D0061234

Strategic Planning for Collegiate Athletics

"**S***trategic Planning for Collegiate Athletics* is a timely and insightful tool for today's athletic administrator. The book encourages quality planning and dissects the process for useful consumption and application. I found Chapter 8, dealing with the planning audit, to be particularly helpful.

In a business where we are driven by *today's* success and *today's* 'hot fires,' we can all use this exceptional text to stimulate, complete, and implement visionary planning."

Robert A. Bowlsby
Director of Athletics,
University of Iowa,
Iowa City

"**I** found this book to be very organized in the presentation of the information. The material is formatted in such a way that athletic administrators can implement either portions or all of the ideas into their departmental plans with ease. Organization and planning for the long range are critical ingredients for the success of the athletics program, given the environment in which intercollegiate athletics finds itself today. This book can give novice administrators an advantage in preparing organizational structures that will be successful for their departments.

The evaluation and audit models at the conclusion of the book will give each reader the opportunity to evaluate the progress that was attained throughout the process and assess where changes will need to be made. We will want to utilize this book in the future as we plan for the success of our athletics program."

Gil Cloud, MS
Director of Intercollegiate Athletics,
Northeastern State University,
Tahlequah, OK

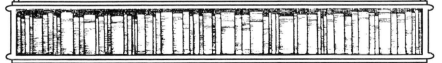

"Strategic Planning for Collegiate Athletics is a welcome addition to practical application-based literature that is central to our industry. Dr. Migliore has taken his expertise on strategic planning and merged it with his love of college athletics to create, along with his worthy co-authors, a book that is not only valuable to practitioners, but that can also be a supplemental text in courses relating to college athletics, sports organizational behavior, and so forth.

In my opinion the approach utilized by the authors is the most valuable contribution of this work. Much of the theory behind what is presented here has been utilized by Migliore in a number of his other works—this book is an application of that work to college athletics. The approach in this work that is intriguing is that each chapter provides an introductory text section that clarifies the concepts related to strategic planning. This section is then followed by a 'workbook' section for each concept of the strategic planning process. This approach is invaluable because it not only ensures that readers understand what they have read, but also provides a medium for application and putting the entire plan together."

William Sutton, EdD
Associate Professor
and Graduate Program Director,
Sport Management Program,
University of Massachusetts
at Amherst

"Strategic Planning for Collegiate Athletics gives both an academic and practical perspective on planning from successful people who have actually done it. Strategic planning often gets put on the back burner, yet it is vital to the future success of any organization. In a thorough and readable way, this book capsulizes the fundamentals of strategic planning into college athletics terminology in a way never done before. This is an extremely useful book, and should be required reading for college athletic administrators."

John D. Swofford, MEd
Commissioner,
Atlantic Coast Conference,
Greensboro, NC

"An exceptional guide with worksheets provided for athletic administrators who wish to lead their departments in determining and realizing their goals. This book provides outstanding useful information and tools for developing a comprehensive strategic plan for success in a variety of athletic areas. In addition, once departments have developed their individualized plans, methods for evaluation and revision are included."

Judy MacLeod, MS
Director of Athletics,
The University of Tulsa,
Oklahoma

Strategic Planning
for Collegiate Athletics

THE HAWORTH PRESS
New, Recent, and Forthcoming Titles
of Related Interest

Strategic Planning for Collegiate Athletics

Deborah A. Yow   R. Henry Migliore

William W. Bowden

Robert E. Stevens   David L. Loudon

Best Business Books
The Haworth Half-Court Press
Imprints of The Haworth Press, Inc.
New York • London • Oxford

Published by

Best Business Books and The Haworth Half-Court Press, imprints of The Haworth Press, Inc., 10 Alice Street, Binghamton, NY 13904-1580

Cover design by Monica L. Seifert.

Library of Congress Cataloging-in-Publication Data

Strategic planning for collegiate athletics / Deborah A. Yow ... [et al.].
    p.   cm.
Includes bibliographical references and index.
ISBN 0-7890-0889-0 (hard) — ISBN 0-7890-1057-7 (pbk.)
1. College sports—Planning. 2. Planning, Strategic. I. Yow, Deborah A.

GV351 .S87 2000   CIP
796'.06'94—dc21   99-055439

CONTENTS

ABOUT THE AUTHORS

Deborah A. Yow, PhD, DHum, is Director of Intercollegiate Athletics at the University of Maryland. She has served as a coach and teacher at the high school and university levels, and began her administrative career as Assistant Director of Gator Boosters at the University of Florida. Dr. Yow was formerly the Associate Director at the University of North Carolina at Greensboro and Director of Intercollegiate Athletics at Saint Louis University. In 1994, she became the first female athletic director in the Atlantic Coast Conference when coming to Maryland. The author of numerous books and articles and a nationally respected speaker, Dr. Yow is a member of the National Collegiate Athletic Association (NCAA) Management Council and other well-known athletic and educational agencies and commissions. In addition, she is President Elect of the National Association of Collegiate Directors of Athletics, a 6,000-member association of athletic administrators representing 1,600 collegiate institutions in North America.

R. Henry Migliore, PhD, is Professor of Strategic Planning and Management at Northeastern State University/Oklahoma State University—Tulsa. Teaching at the collegiate level for 30 years, he has taught undergraduate and graduate courses and assisted in executive education at Northeastern State University, Oklahoma State University, Oral Roberts University, Texas A&M, Pepperdine, Central Michigan, ITESM Campus Guadalajara, and the University of Calgary. The author of over 80 articles and numerous books, Dr. Migliore serves as a consultant to athletic programs across the United States.

William W. Bowden, EdD, PhD, is founder and president of Strategic Management Consultants, a firm that has worked with dozens of colleges, universities, corporations, and the National Collegiate Athletic Association (NCAA) in relation to their athletic interests and management challenges. The author of more than 30 research reports, articles, and books, Dr. Bowden also served as a teacher and administrator at the university level for 17 years.

Robert E. Stevens, PhD, MBA, is Professor of Marketing in the College of Business at The University of Louisiana at Monroe. He is the author of 16 books and more than 120 articles dealing with marketing and its application to various areas. Dr. Stevens has served as a consultant to local, regional, and national firms for research projects, feasibility studies, and marketing planning, and was a partner in a marketing research company for three years prior to moving to Louisiana. He also taught for ten years at Oral Roberts University, where has was active in marketing projects for the university and ministry. Dr. Stevens is a member of the Southwest Marketing Association, the Southern Marketing Association, and the Atlantic Marketing Association.

David L. Loudon, PhD, MBA, is Head of the Department of Management and Marketing in the College of Business at The University of Louisiana at Monroe. He is the author of over 50 articles and 8 books on consumer behavior and legal services marketing. Dr. Loudon has conducted research in the United States, Europe, and Latin America on a variety of topics, including the application of marketing concepts to nontraditional areas. He has served as a consultant to numerous organizations and is president of a computer software firm. Dr. Loudon is also a member of the Southwest Marketing Association, the Southern Marketing Association, the Atlantic Marketing Association, and the American Marketing Association.

Preface

This book is primarily designed for administrators and other practicing professionals associated with collegiate as well as high school and recreational athletics and sports programs. It will also serve as a supplemental text for college courses on sports/athletics administration and planning (with the general principles being applicable to administration, management, and planners in other fields).

We had three primary considerations when preparing this book. The first was length. Our goal was to discuss the topics and issues that are most relevant and practical, thus limiting the scope and size of the book to allow for timely reading and application. As a result, we had to omit numerous topics and provide a somewhat succinct discussion of others. The essential concepts and techniques are presented in a focused and concise form.

The second consideration was to present material that was theoretically sound but also readily applicable in college, university, and other athletics environments—and therefore immediately useful for decision making in those settings. We have also included worksheets at the end of each chapter to help readers develop their own strategic plans.

The final consideration was to provide a set of appendixes to illustrate various aspects of strategic planning and a sample strategic plan. Thus, the reader not only can read about strategic planning but can actually see what one looks like. This is useful in evaluating plans prepared by others or in preparing your own.

The end result, we believe, is a book that is both readable and readily applicable by those involved with athletics and sports administration.

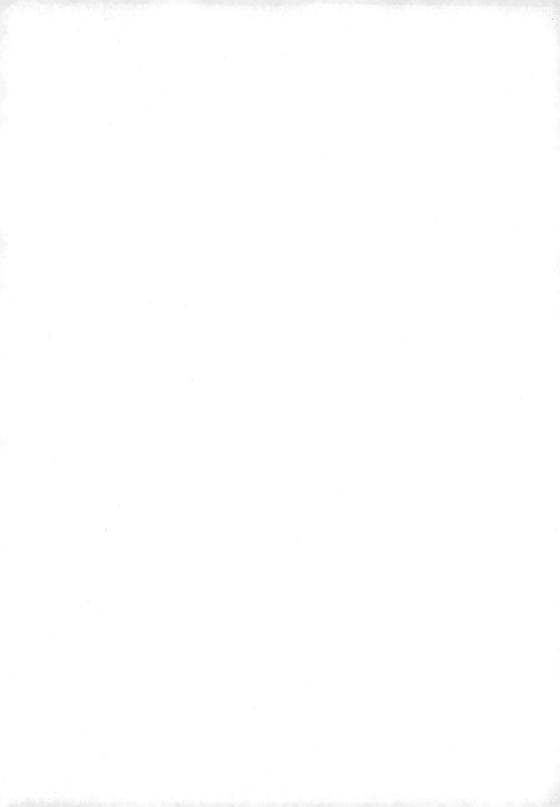

Acknowledgments

A book is seldom the work of the authors alone, but involves the efforts of a great number of people. Among those who were of considerable help in the process of preparing this manuscript were: Joyce Taylor, who tirelessly typed drafts of the manuscript; the Department of Intercollegiate Athletics at the University of Maryland, which served as a benign laboratory as well as a lens through which issues were frequently viewed; and Rashmi Sane, for typing the final version of the manuscript.

Chapter 1

Perspectives on Planning
for Athletics Programs

Many athletics departments are struggling to succeed. For some, survival is their main issue. Clearly, every university and college with athletics programs is looking for ways to adapt to a changing environment. If you are challenged with any of the following issues or questions, this book will be important to you.

- Why is there sometimes confusion among our athletics staff regarding what we are trying to accomplish?
- Why is there an unacceptable level of turnover of people in our intercollegiate athletics department, including leadership positions?
- How can we make more effective use of our human, financial, and facility resources? How can we better empower and enable our valued employees?
- As a person in leadership, why am I working twelve hours a day and yet, cannot keep up?
- Why have we not had the success we expected and needed on a number of projects and initiatives?
- What are the internal and external factors that are keys to our expected level of success?
- Why have many among the boosters, donors, and members of the university community viewed our purpose and our activities as largely without merit or significance?
- Why does our department lack enthusiasm, a team spirit, and a sense of mission?

If you are contending with one of these or similar issues that may be inducing stress in your life, the answer might be that your department lacks sound long-term strategic planning (Yow, Bowden, and Humphrey, 1998). An important part of strategic planning is the team-building approach of developing leaders and involving a broad range of people in the plan.

PLANNING IS IMPORTANT

Planning as a part of the management process is crucial to the success of any organization (Bridges and Roquemore, 1992). This is especially true for college and university athletics departments, although insufficient research has been done on the relationship of planning to successful athletics departments. In 1998, however, a study of the relationship between the use of the planning process and athletics departments' effectiveness was conducted by Bowden and Yow among a selected group of athletics departments. The study found that:

- Comprehensive, better-funded, and generally respected athletics programs were more frequently engaged in formal planning than other athletics programs.
- A majority of these departments had been using strategic, long-range planning for less than eight years.
- Departmental effectiveness was increased by the presence of written yearly and long-range plans, when those plans were followed and executed carefully.
- The lack of a written plan (yearly and/or long-range) hindered the ability of the athletics program to generate consistent support, achieve at desired levels in programs and services, and maintain its desired image among its numerous publics.

One of the most important conclusions drawn from this study is that systematic and careful planning is an integral function within athletics departments that (1) make the most effective use of resources and (2) achieve at consistently high levels nationally in the important categories of competitive results, academic outcomes (graduation rates), student athlete welfare, facilities enhancement, fund-raising, and other strategic outcomes (Bowden and Yow, 1998).

Of the large number of decisions made by an athletics department or by individual administrators, there are a handful that can significantly impact the direction and future of the athletics program. These strategic decisions require careful identification and thoughtful consideration. This is the nature of the role of strategic planning.

Perspectives of strategic thinking can be illustrated with this question: Who are the two most important persons responsible for the success of an airplane's flight? Typical responses would be:

- the pilot and the navigator,
- the pilot and the maintenance supervisor,
- the pilot and the air traffic controller, or
- the pilot and the flight engineer.

All of the responses recognize the day-to-day, hands-on importance of the pilot—and they all introduce one of several other important support or auxiliary functionaries to the answer. However, each of these segmented responses ignores the one person who is perhaps the single most important individual for the ultimate success of the airplane—the designer. The pilot and the designer are perhaps the two most important individuals for the success of an airplane: A pilot because of his or her day-to-day responsibilities in commanding the craft, and the designer because of his or her ability to create a concept that can be economically constructed, easily operated by any normally competent flight crew, and maintained safely by the ground crew.

Most Athletic Directors probably perceive themselves as the "pilot" of the department: taking off, landing, conferring with the navigator, and communicating with the air traffic controller. Athletic Directors generally view themselves as the chief hands-on operational manager. However, what has been most lacking in athletics departments has been an appreciation for the strategic viewpoint. There is a need for more emphasis on the "designer's" approach to operating the athletics department. A well-conceived strategic planning system can facilitate this emphasis. This emphasis will include a long-term focus when devising the plans. This will provide steady, longitudinal direction to any athletics program (Yow and Bowden, 1998).

WHAT IS PLANNING?

Planning may be defined as a managerial activity that involves analyzing the environment, setting objectives, deciding on specific actions needed to reach the objectives, and also providing feedback on results. This *process* should be distinguished from the plan itself, which is a written document containing the results of the planning process; it is a written statement of what is to be done and how it is to be done. Planning is a continuous process that both precedes and follows other functions, in which plans are made and executed, and results are used to make new plans as the process continues.

TYPES OF PLANS

There are many types of plans, but most can be categorized as *strategic* or *tactical*. Strategic plans cover a longer period of time and may be referred to as *long-term* plans. They are broad in scope and basically answer the question of how an organization is to commit its resources over the next five to ten years. Strategic plans are altered as needed to reflect changes in the environment or overall direction of the athletics department.

Tactical plans cover a short time period, usually a year or less. They are often referred to as *short-term* or *operational* plans. They specify what is to be done in a given year to move the organization toward its long-term objectives. In other words, what you do this year (short term) needs to be tied to where you want to be five to ten years in the future (long term).

To a great extent, athletics departments that have been involved in planning have focused on short-term rather than long-term planning. Although this is better than not planning at all, it also means each year's plan is not related to anything long-term in nature and often fails to move the organization toward its preferred future.

Departmental units and individual events of the athletic department require planning. A departmental unit encompasses a large set of activities involving a whole area of a department's capabilities, such as planning for and carrying out the academic assistance program for student athletes (tutors, study tables, counseling, monitoring academic progress, recognition of achievements, etc.).

Planning for the range of activities within the department's units involves:

1. Dividing the total set of activities into meaningful parts.
2. Assigning planning responsibility for each part to appropriate people.
3. Assigning target dates for completion of plans.
4. Determining and allocating the resources needed for each part.

Each major unit within an athletics department should have a strategic plan in place to provide a blueprint for the unit over time. Moreover, the plan of each unit should be integrally tied to the department's overall strategic plan.

A departmental *event* is generally of less scope and complexity. An event may be a part of a broader program or it may be self-contained and require the coordinated efforts of a number of units. Even though it is a special or a one-time event, planning is essential to accomplishing the objectives of the project and coordinating the activities that make up the event. A plan to host a conference or NCAA championship event, or have a "Walk, Run, Roll" sponsored fund-raising event for women's athletics teams, or a "Friends of Athletics Day" on campus would be examples of a project plan.

ADVANTAGES OF PLANNING FOR ATHLETICS DEPARTMENTS

Why should an athletics department devote time to planning? Consider the following questions:

- Do you know where you are going and how you are going to get there?
- Does each person associated with the athletics department know what you as a department are trying to accomplish?
- Do all those involved know what is expected of them?

If the answer to any of these is no, then your athletics program needs to develop a strategic long-range plan with as many people involved as possible in the preparation of the plan.

In many small departments, administrators or staff members may object to planning, thinking that it makes no sense for them, since theirs is only a small organization and everyone in the department knows what happened in the past year and what is likely to happen in the coming year. Another frequent objection is that there is no time for planning. A third is that there are not enough resources to allow for planning.

All of these objections actually point out the necessity for planning, even in the small department. Such an organization may actually have a sizable budget, making it imperative to have a plan of where the department is heading. The observation that there is no time for planning may seem accurate, but this is probably due to the lack of planning in the past, which has left insufficient time for attention to such necessities. Finally, the argument that there are insufficient resources actually justifies the role of planning in order to obtain the maximum benefit from those resources being used in the department. Thus, planning is a critical element for the success of any athletics department.

Planning has many advantages. For example, it helps athletics department administrators to adapt to changing environments, take advantage of opportunities created by change, reach agreements on major issues, and place responsibility more precisely. It also gives a sense of direction to staff members as well as providing a basis for gaining their commitment. The sense of vision that can be provided in a well-written plan also instills a sense of loyalty in those associated with the athletics department.

An athletics department can benefit from the planning process because this systematic, continuing process allows it to achieve the following:

1. Assess the department's market position. This involves what is termed a SWOT analysis—examining the department's internal **S**trengths and **W**eaknesses and external **O**pportunities and **T**hreats. Without explicit planning, these elements may go unrecognized.
2. Establish goals, objectives, priorities, and strategies to be completed within specified time periods. Planning will enable the department to assess accomplishment of the goals that are set

and will help motivate staff to work together to achieve shared goals.

3. Achieve greater staff commitment and teamwork aimed at meeting challenges and solving problems presented by changing conditions.

4. Muster its resources to meet these changes through anticipation and preparation. "Adapt or diminish" is a very accurate admonition.

Administrators cannot control the future, but they should attempt to identify and isolate present actions and forecast how results can be expected to influence the future. The primary purpose of planning, then, is to ensure that current programs can be used to increase the chances of achieving future objectives and goals; that is, to increase the chances of making better decisions today that affect tomorrow's performance.

Unless planning leads to improved performance, it is not worthwhile. Thus, to have an athletics department that looks forward to the future and tries to stay alive and prosper in a changing environment, there must be active, vigorous, continuous, and creative planning. Otherwise, a department will find itself in the untenable position of simply reacting to its immediate environment.

There are basically two reasons for planning: (1) protective benefits resulting from reduced chances for error in decision making, and (2) positive benefits in the form of increased success in reaching departmental objectives.

Often, when athletics departments plan poorly, they must constantly devote their energies to solving problems that would not have existed, or at least would be much less serious, with planning. They spend their time fighting fires rather than practicing fire prevention.

Long-range planning can become a means of renewal in the life of a department if the following points are remembered:

1. A unified purpose can be achieved only when all segments of the life of the department see themselves as part of a larger whole, with a single goal.

2. Isolated individual decisions and commitments often influence future plans, even when they are not intended to do so.

3. When careful planning is lacking, competition among groups and duplication of effort result.
4. Coordinated planning gives a sense of perspective in relation to the mission of the department as a whole.

PLANNING'S PLACE IN THE ATHLETICS PROGRAM

All administrators and indeed all staff members in the athletics department engage in planning to some degree. As a general rule, the larger the athletics program becomes the more the primary planning activities become associated with groups of people as opposed to individuals.

Some larger departments develop a planning committee or staff. Organizations set up such a planning group for one or more of the following reasons.

1. *Planning takes time.* A planning group can reduce the workload of individual staff within the department.
2. *Planning takes coordination.* A planning group can help integrate and coordinate the planning activities of individual staff.
3. *Planning takes expertise.* A planning group can bring to a particular problem more tools and techniques than any single individual within the athletics department.
4. *Planning takes objectivity.* A planning group can take a broader view than one individual and go beyond specific projects and particular athletics department units.

A planning group generally has three basic areas of responsibility. First, it assists the department in developing goals, policies, and strategies for the athletics program. The group facilitates the planning process by scanning and monitoring the department's environment. A second major responsibility of the group is to coordinate the planning of different levels and units within the department. Finally, the planning group acts as an organizational resource for Athletic Administrators and other staff who lack expertise in planning.

In smaller departments, planning and execution are usually carried out by the same people. The greatest challenge is to set aside time for planning in the midst of the other day-to-day activities.

RESISTANCE TO THE PLANNING PROCESS

There are three main reasons why planning does not get done in athletics programs today: (1) administrators lack training, (2) some perceive it as unnecessary and therefore an unjustifiable addition to their workload, and (3) problems in implementation.

Lack of Management Training

Many Athletic Administrators have a minimumn amount of management or administrative training and often are placed in their position without significant or meaningful experience in administration. As a result, the planning, objective setting, and other superordinate management functions are sometimes neglected or inadequately performed.

Planning Is Perceived As Unnecessary

The reluctance to plan stems from the fact that many departments view the application of strategic planning as unnecessary. Some have felt that because athletics departments are part of a college or university setting that they are not businesses—and therefore should not be required to pursue formal, systematic long-range and strategic planning as would occur in a well-run business.

Although strategic planning has received increasing recognition for its applicability to athletics departments, there remain some administrators who doubt its worth to an athletics department.

Conversely, there is increasingly a new breed of Athletic Administrator taking his or her place in athletics departments across the United States. These leaders are committed to using all the effective management tools available to them in administering their departments and units within their athletics departments, including the use of systematic, careful planning to make the most effective use of resources to achieve worthy goals.

In addition, the relatively new NCAA Certification Program for athletics departments requires an approach to management and planning that embodies the integral function of strategic long-range planning.

Implementation Problems

Although there is much academic and theoretical support for planning, the actual implementation of it often runs aground on the shores of departmental reality. Even among very progressive athletics programs one sometimes finds significant resistance to planning. Some of the most common arguments against it are:

1. Planning is not action oriented.
2. Planning takes too much time; we are too busy to plan.
3. Planning is unrealistic because of the rapid change in our environment (demographics, professional sports teams, etc.).
4. Planning becomes an end, not just a means to an end.

Many of these arguments result from the same kind of thinking that would rank the pilot as the only important person in the success of an airplane. To be helpful, planning does not depend on complete forecasting accuracy. In fact, a variety of futuristic alternatives or scenarios can be very helpful in establishing planning parameters. Often a best-case, most likely case, and worst-case approach is used. This three-level forecast gives dimension to the process of recognizing, anticipating, and managing change.

The objection that planning is not "hands-on" and related to the important day-to-day operations of the department is frequent. However, this point of view is shortsighted in terms of long-term success. Planning is not just for dreamers; in fact, it lets the department's administrative team determine what can be done today to accomplish or avoid some future circumstance.

Planning sometimes becomes an end in the minds of some users. This is particularly true when planning is solely a committee responsibility within an athletics program. A committee staff can facilitate the strategic planning process, but the process will not be a dynamic life-blood activity of the organization without the ongoing involvement of a wide range of staff members. President Eisenhower has been widely quoted as saying, "Plans are nothing; planning is everything." The belief he expressed was that the actual plan itself was not the end, but that the process of planning/developing futuristic scenarios, evaluating the environment and competition, assessing internal strengths and capabilities, and revising objectives and tactics was the organization dialogue that was most important. This department dialogue ideally breaks down barriers to communication, exposes blind spots, tests logic, measures the environment, and determines feasibility. The end result is more effective and efficient implementation of departmental activity.

The advantages of planning far outweigh any of the previously stated and other perceived disadvantages. Planning not only should be done, but must be done, in order for an athletics program to achieve optimum success.

THE GREATEST NEEDS OF TODAY'S ATHLETICS PROGRAMS

In informal surveys of athletics programs, administrators were reasonably sure that strategic planning is important. To put matters into perspective, let us try to translate athletics department success into a formula:

$$X = f (a,b,c,d,e,f,g,h,i \ldots)$$

In this case X is success for the athletics department, a dependent variable, and is on the left side of the equation. The $=$ sign means a balance, or equal to what is on the other side; the f means "function of." On the right side are all the independent variables that affect success:

a. Quality and effectiveness of departmental leadership
b. View of the role of athletics as related to the mission and purpose of the institution (as held by the college of university community—including alumni, and by the plenary staff of the athletics department itself)
c. Planning system
d. Organization system
e. Control system
f. Quality of customer service (internal and external customers)
g. Funding level
h. Conference affiliation
i. Location

    j. Capacity of athletics facilities

    k. Other variables

Only a few independent variables are listed, but the possibilities are endless. The most consistent among integral variables is the function of planning. Indeed, effective planning appears to be among the three most important variables present in highly achieving athletics programs.

When planning is given appropriate priority in athletics programs, lack of direction and inefficiency were far less common than in the 32 percent of programs surveyed where consistent, sound planning was not recognized as preeminently integral to the success of the department.

The educational, societal, and sheer human impact of athletics programs, along with the complex conditions of their internal and external operational culture, mandate that an athletics department have the discipline and good management sense to plan carefully. In addition, the sobering financial, student athlete welfare, academic, and organizational challenges of a new millennium are already being felt in college and university athletics programs throughout the United States.

SUMMARY

In this chapter, we have attempted to establish our belief that (1) methods used successfully in numerous businesses and organizations are applicable to athletics departments; (2) there is an important place for better planning and management; (3) many Athletic Administrators do believe that there is a need for planning; (4) one of the most compelling needs in athletics programs is the need to overcome the resistance to planning and begin to carry out that function effectively, and (5) all sound management models include an integral place for the role of effective planning.

The philosophy of this book is that for everyone in the athletics department to be successful, a strategic plan is essential. Throughout years of professional employment in athletics and consulting with athletics programs, the authors have observed that with sound planning you can expect the following:

1. A sense of enthusiasm in your athletics department.
2. A five-year plan in writing to which most everyone is committed.
3. A sense of commitment by the entire department to its overall direction.
4. Clear job duties and responsibilities.
5. Time for the leaders to do what they can most effectively do for the athletics program.
6. Clear and evident improvement in the effectiveness of each staff member.
7. The ability to measure very specifically the growth and contribution made by the leaders and other staff members at the close of their careers in the department.
8. Guaranteed leadership of the athletics program because a plan is in place in writing and is understood. Even more important, a management team and philosophy will be in place to guide the department into its next era of growth.

In the next chapter, we present an overview of the entire strategic planning process (see also Appendix A for a complete outline for constructing a strategic plan). In subsequent chapters we discuss each step of the planning process. We explain the theory behind each part and give actual examples to help you understand that step. Appendixes B and C provide samples of strategic plans. Make notes on your own situation as you read. Read on with anticipation.

Chapter 2

Overview of Strategic Planning

In this chapter, we present an overview of the strategic planning process. Each of the areas discussed is examined in considerably more detail in later chapters. Our intention here is to provide an introduction to the major components of the process of strategic planning.

WHAT IS STRATEGIC PLANNING?

The word strategic means "pertaining to strategy." Strategy is derived from the Greek word *strategia*, which means generalship, art of the general or, more broadly, leadership. The word "strategic," when used in the context of planning, provides a perspective to planning that is long-term in nature and deals with achieving specified end results. In comparison, as military strategy has as its objective the winning of a war, and strategic planning has as its objective the achievement of departmental goals.

Strategic decisions must be differentiated from tactical decisions, however. Strategic decisions outline the overall game plan or approach, while tactical decisions involve implementing various activities that are necessary to carry out a strategy. For example, an athletics program that decides to change conference affiliation is making a strategic decision. Many other decisions must then be made regarding whether or not to become an independent athletics program or affiliate with another athletics conference, and if so, which available conference. This has long-term implications and is therefore strategic in nature.

Other decisions must be made relating to (a) funding for possible increased team travel costs, (b) preparing for income changes resulting from new revenue-sharing formulas that differ from conference to conference, (c) changes in the student athlete initial eligibility and continuing eligibility requirements that vary from conference to conference, and (d) other issues. Indeed, intercollegiate Athletic Administrators/Planners sometimes find that the tactical and implementational steps are not practical or even possible for the department (or may not be philosophically tenable) and therefore that the strategic initiative is not feasible during the term of the current plan. These are tactical decisions needed to carry out or implement the previous strategic decision. Thus, the strategic decision provides the overall framework within which the tactical decisions are made. It is critically important that administrators are able to differentiate between these types of decisions to identify whether the decisions have short- or long-term implications.

THE STRATEGIC PLANNING PROCESS IN ATHLETICS

The strategic planning process is basically a matching process involving the department's resources and opportunities. The objective of this process is to peer through the "strategic window" (an opportunity that may have a relatively short shelf life) and identify opportunities that the individual department is equipped to take advantage of or respond to. Thus the strategic management process can be defined as a managerial process that involves matching departmental capabilities to departmental opportunities. These opportunities are created over time and decisions revolve around investing or divesting resources to address these opportunities. The context in which these strategic decisions are made is: (a) the department's operating environment, (b) the department's purpose or mission, and (c) its objectives. This overall process is depicted in Figure 2.1. Strategic planning is the process that ties all these elements together to facilitate strategic choices that are consistent with all three areas and then implements and evaluates these choices. Appendix A presents an outline of a strategic plan.

The successful results of planning described earlier in this chapter can be achieved through implementing an effective strategic plan-

FIGURE 2.1. The Strategic Planning Process

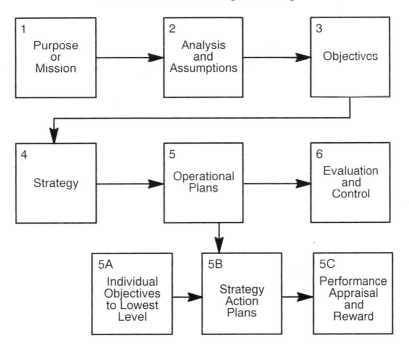

ning process (Bradford and Cohen, 1984, p. 258). The following breakdown of this process is a complete outline of the system capable of creating authentic change in the attitudes of personnel as well as in productivity. Such a philosophy involves:

1. Defining a department's purpose and reason for being.
2. Analyzing the environment in which it operates, realistically assessing its strengths and weaknesses, and making assumptions about unpredictable future events. The environment would include the department's institutional setting as well as its city, state, and region, along with its conference milieu.
3. Prescribing written, specific, and measurable objectives in principal result areas contributing to the department's purpose.
4. Developing strategies for how to use available resources to reach objectives.

5. Developing operational plans to meet objectives, including establishing individual objectives and strategies.
6. Evaluating performance to determine whether it is keeping pace with attainment of objectives and is consistent with defined purpose and changing objectives, strategies, or operational plans in light of the evaluation.

It is important to recognize at this point what we call "the two observable Ps." The first P means *product*—get the plan in writing. The plan must be something you can hold in your hand, a written observable product of your efforts. If the plan is not in writing, it is called daydreaming. When it is in writing, you are indicating to yourself and others that you are serious about it. The second P represents *process*—every plan must have maximum input from everyone. Those who execute the plan must be involved in construction of the plan. The best way to ensure failure in planning is to overlook either the product or the process. They are equally important.

While there are many different ways in which an athletics department can approach the strategic planning process, a systematic approach that carries the organization through a series of integral steps helps to focus attention on a basic set of questions each organization must answer:

1. *What will we do?* This question focuses attention on the specific needs which the department will try to meet.
2. *For whom will we do it?* This question addresses the need for a department to identify the various groups whose needs will be met.
3. *How will we do what we want to do?* Answering this question forces the organization to think about the many avenues through which service and activities may be channeled.

The strategic planning process used by an athletics department will require departmental leadership to deal with these questions on a continuing basis. The department evolves over time into what its mission and purpose calls for it to be and therefore into what it was established to be, to do the work that only it can do.

In summary, strategic planning involves the following steps:

1. Defining an organization's purpose and reason for being.
2. Analyzing the environment, assessing its strengths and weaknesses, and making assumptions.
3. Prescribing written, specific, and measurable objectives in the principal result areas that contribute to the organization's purpose.
4. Developing strategies on how to use available resources to meet objectives.
5. Developing operational plans to meet objectives, including plans for all individuals in the organization.
6. Setting up control and evaluation procedures to determine if performance is keeping pace with attainment of objectives and if it is consistent with defined purpose.

The six steps of the strategic planning process, as illustrated in Figure 2.1, are important because they force the organization to consider certain essential questions. As each step requires the people at various organizational levels to discuss, study, and negotiate, the process as a whole fosters a planning mentality. When the six steps are completed, the result is a strategic plan specifying why the organization exists, what it is trying to accomplish, and how resources will be utilized to accomplish objectives and fulfill its purpose.

Defining Purpose

The first and perhaps the most important consideration when developing a strategic plan is to define the purpose, mission, or the "reason for being" of the organization or any specific part of it. This is usually a difficult process even though it may appear simple. For example, an athletics department that defines itself as "a functioning unit that is successful in its competitive outcomes" may be on the right track, but will constantly face the need to further define and expand upon this definition. What considerations are important to the department other than winning or losing athletics events? At what level, in general, would competitive outcomes need to be for "success" to have been achieved? Other issues and questions related to the comprehensive purpose for the department should be addressed. Granted these elements may change as an athletics department evolves and grows; but thinking through these issues provides a sense of vision and also prevents the department from pursuing activities that do not fit in with what the department wants to do or be.

The staff of the department should try to visualize what they want the organization to become, and should incorporate this dream or vision into their purpose statement. If they can see where they are going and have an image of the real mission of the organization, their plans will come into focus more easily. A vision of what can be accomplished creates the spark, energy, and imagination for the whole planning and management process. It is important to spend ample time defining this purpose statement. The process should emphasize involving everyone in the vision of how things can be. Without a vision for the department and therefore for their work, employees of the athletics department tend to function without the teamwork, sustained commitments, goals, and productivity that would otherwise be possible.

A good statement of purpose not only clarifies what the department does, it sets boundaries. It defines what the department will not do. It helps limit expectations, and that alone can make it a helpful tool.

Analysis and Assumptions

It is also important for the athletics department to gauge the environment within which it operates. The only way we can manage change effectively is to constantly monitor the environment within which we operate. This analysis stage is where we look at the external environment, internal strengths and weaknesses, and potential threats and opportunities (Oakley and Krug, 1991, p. 34).

Many organizations have found it useful to use an analysis framework referred to earlier as a SWOT analysis. SWOT is an acronym for strengths, weaknesses, opportunities, and threats: strengths and weaknesses refer to elements internal to the organization, while opportunities and threats are external to the organization. A detailed SWOT analysis helps the department take a good look at the organization's favorable and unfavorable factors with a view toward building on strengths and eliminating or minimizing weaknesses. At the same time, the department must also access external opportunities that could be pursued and threats that must be dealt with in order for the department to survive.

The next stage is to state your major assumptions about spheres over which you have little or absolutely no control, such as the external environment. One good place to start is to extend some of the items studied in the external analysis. Should this stage appear relatively unimportant in developing a strategic plan, consider that by *not* making explicit assumptions you are making one major implicit assumption—things are going to remain the same and most things that happen are either not strategically important or will not affect the department. In intercollegiate athletics, as in most fields, this is a false and very dangerous assumption.

Establishing Objectives

Often the words "key results," "goals," and "targets" are used synonymously with objectives. Think about an archer drawing an arrow and aiming directly at a target. The bull's-eye represents exactly where you want to be at a certain point in time. An Athletic Director wants the entire department aimed at the same target just as an archer wants the arrow aimed at the target. At the other extreme, an archer who shoots arrows off in any direction is liable to hit almost anything—including the wrong target. People get confused and disorganized if they do not know where they are going.

Objectives must be clear, concise, written statements outlining what is to be accomplished in key priority areas, over a certain time period, in measurable terms that are consistent with the overall purpose of the organization. Objectives can be classified as routine, problem solving, innovative, team, personal, or budget performance. Objectives do not determine the future, but they are the means by which the resources and energies are mobilized for the shaping of the future.

Objectives are the results that are desired upon completion of the planning period. In the absence of objectives, no sense of direction can be attained in decision making. In other words, if you do not know where you are going, any road will take you there. In planning, objectives answer one of the basic questions posed in the planning process: Where do we want to go? These objectives become the focal point for strategy decisions.

Another basic purpose served by objectives is in the evaluation of performance. Objectives in the strategic plan become the achievement goals used for this evaluation. It is impossible to evaluate performance without some standard against which results can be compared. The objectives become the standards for evaluation because they are the statement of results desired by the planner.

Strategy Development

After developing a set of objectives for the time period covered by the strategic plan, a strategy to accomplish those objectives must be formulated. An overall strategy must first be designed; then the operational strategies must be developed.

Strategy alternatives are the alternate courses of action evaluated by management before a commitment is made to specific options outlined in the strategic plan. Listed under *each* objective are the specific strategies or actions that must be carried out to achieve that objective. Thus, strategy is the link between objectives and results.

Operational Plans

After all the steps have been taken and a strategy has been developed to meet the athletics department's objectives and goals, it is time to develop an operational or action plan. The operational plan stage is the "action" or "doing" stage. Here you hire, enable, terminate, build, advertise, and so on. How many times has a group of people planned something, gotten enthusiastic, and then nothing happened? This is usually because they did not complete an operational or action plan to implement their strategy.

Operational plans must be developed for all the areas that are used to support the overall strategy. These include production, communication, finance, and staffing. Each plan is designed to spell out what needs to happen in a given area to implement the strategic plan.

Supporting the operational plans are the individual plans of all members of the department. These are shown as steps 5A, 5B, and 5C in Figure 2.1. When planning is carried out from the top to the lowest level in the organization, everyone becomes involved in setting and negotiating personal objectives which support the organization's objectives. Then each person begins to develop an individual action plan that is used to accomplish these personal objectives. Finally, the personnel performance appraisal, which must be done on an individual basis, uses individual objectives as the basis of appraisal and reward. In some settings, the performance appraisal is better carried out as part of the sixth and final step, "Evaluation and Control."

Evaluation and Control

Failure to establish procedures to appraise and control the strategic plan can lead to less than optimal performance. A plan is not complete until the controls are identified and the procedures for recording and transmitting control information to the administrators of the plan are established. Many organizations fail to understand the importance of establishing procedures to appraise and control the planning process. Control should be a natural follow-through in developing a plan.

Planning and control should be integral processes. The strategic planning process results in a strategic plan. This plan is implemented (activities are performed in the manner described in the plan) and results are produced. These results are wins/losses, graduation rates, fund-raising results, etc. Information on these and other key result areas is provided to administrators, who compare the results with objectives to evaluate performance. This performance evaluation identifies the areas where decisions must be made to adjust activities, add staff, or adjust financial resources allocated. The actual decision making controls the plan by altering it in a manner to accomplish stated objectives, and a new cycle begins.

STRATEGIC PLANNING AS A PROCESS

The word "process" refers to a series of actions directed toward prescribed outcomes. The actions are the activities in which the department engages to accomplish objectives and fulfill its mission. There are several important reasons for viewing strategic planning as a process. First, a change in any component of the process will affect most or all of the other components. For example, a change in purpose or objective will lead to new analysis, strategies, and evaluations. Thus, major changes that affect the department must lead to a reevaluation of all the elements of the plan.

A second reason for viewing strategic planning as a process is that a process can be studied and improved. An athletics program that is just getting involved in strategic planning will need to review the whole process on an annual basis, not only to account for changing environmental forces, but also to improve or refine the plan. Purpose statements, objectives, strategies, and appraisal techniques can be fine-tuned over time as the planners gain more experience and as new and better information becomes available.

Finally and perhaps most important, involvement in the strategic planning process can become the vehicle through which the whole organization mobilizes its energies to accomplish its purpose. If all members of an organization can participate in the process in some way, an atmosphere can be created within the organization that implies that doing the right things and doing things right is everybody's job. In an athletics department this produces a culture of success. Participation instills ownership. It's not "my plan" or "their plan," but "our plan" that becomes important; and everyone will want to make a contribution to make it happen.

STRATEGY IMPLEMENTATION

The focus of this book is on the strategic planning process that results in the development of a strategic plan. This plan becomes the blueprint for carrying out the many activities in which an athletics program is involved. There are many other issues that determine the effectiveness of an organization that are beyond the scope of this book. These issues essentially revolve around implementing the strategic plan through (1) staffing and training personnel and volunteers, (2) developing organizational relationships among staff, (3) achieving commitment, (4) developing a positive organizational culture, (5) leadership styles, and (6) personnel evaluation and reward systems.

There is a wise saying that indicates, "where there is no vision, the people perish." It is also true that without people, especially the right people, the vision will perish. Both effective planning and implementation are needed to create an effective athletics department. The strategic plan concentrates on "doing the right things" while implementation concentrates on "doing things right." An example of a brief strategic plan for an athletics department is presented in Appendix B.

SUMMARY

In this chapter we have presented an overview of the strategic planning process in which a series of thought-provoking questions must be answered. The process is a set of integral steps that carry the planners through a sequence that involves providing answers to these questions and then continually rethinking and reevaluating these answers as the athletics department and its environment change.

A helpful tool at this stage is the "Planning Process Worksheet" that follows. This worksheet, when thoughtfully filled out, will help you get the planning process started in your department. It will establish the planning parameters to improve the efficiency and effectiveness of the department.

PLANNING PROCESS WORKSHEET

This worksheet is provided to aid the athletics department in starting the strategic planning process.

1. Who should be involved in the planning process?

   _____

   _____

   _____

   _____

2. Where will planning sessions be held?

   _____

   _____

   _____

   _____

3. When will planning sessions be held?

   _____

   _____

   _____

   _____

4. What types of background material do participants need prior to starting the first session?

   _____

   _____

   _____

   _____

5. Who will lead the process? Who will ultimately be responsible for arranging sessions and getting material typed, reproduced, and distributed?

_____

_____

_____

_____

6. When and how will members of the staff and others be involved in the process?

_____

_____

_____

_____

7. How will the results be communicated to everyone in the organization?

_____

_____

_____

_____

8. Who will train/supervise staff members in working with their own staff and volunteers in setting objectives, developing action plans, and performance appraisals?

_____

_____

_____

_____

9. How frequently will the process be reviewed and by whom?

_____

_____

_____

_____

10. Who will be responsible for interfacing with external groups (the university community, the faculty athletics committee, boards, the NCAA and other agencies, the local and national sports media, and other entities) in preparing the plan?

_____

_____

_____

_____

Chapter 3

Defining Your Purpose

This chapter outlines the first step in the strategic planning process. Without a clear and carefully considered statement of purpose all other stages of the process will be misguided. We will therefore discuss the value of defining the department's purpose and describe how to write effective statements of purpose or mission. Also, examples of mission statements are provided for an athletics department as a whole, as well as sample mission statements for individual units within an athletics department.

THE IMPORTANCE OF DEFINING PURPOSE

The first and probably most important consideration when developing a strategic plan is to define the purpose, mission, or "reason for being" for the organization or any specific part of it. This is usually a difficult process. Peter Drucker, a management consultant and writer, has led the way in emphasizing the importance of defining purpose. An organization develops to satisfy a need in the marketplace. Drucker states that the organization's purpose is defined by the need that the customer satisfies by buying a product or service. Thus, satisfying the customer is the mission and purpose of every business. Organizations need a clear definition of purpose and mission. This raises the questions "What is our purpose?" and "What should it be?" Drucker's answer is that only a clear definition of the mission and purpose of the business makes possible clear and realistic business objectives. It is the foundation for priorities, strategies, plans, and work assignments. It is the starting point for the design of managerial structure and jobs (Drucker, 1974).

Clearly, if purpose is defined casually or introspectively, or if the list of key result areas neglects some of the less obvious threats and opportunities, the organization is at risk. As Calvin Coolidge put it: "No enterprise can exist for itself alone. It ministers to some great need, it performs some great service not for itself but for others; or failing therein it ceases to be profitable and ceases to exist."

It is in the purpose statement that the vision for the athletics program must be reflected. This purpose statement sets the stage for all planning. Objectives, which are covered later in the text, must by their very nature contribute to achieving what is in the purpose statement. Unfortunately, it is the case that for individuals and educational institutions, these enabling objectives are often missing. For example, in a study of a selected group of college and university administrations, it was discovered that 85 percent of those surveyed had some form of a purpose and mission statement, but only about 50 percent had *specific and measurable* objectives of what was to be accomplished. A random study of 260 adults ages nineteen to sixty-seven found that 217 could cite at least one identified, definitive personal goal; but only 167 could identify at least one specific enabling objective to be achieved in order to reach their goals (Bowden and Yow, 1996).

A mission statement aids an athletics department by the following enabling features:

1. Giving it a reason for being.
2. Defining what it will and will not do.
3. Describing the needs the department is attempting to meet.
4. Giving a general description of how the organization is going to respond to that need.
5. Serve as a basis for developing objectives.
6. Helping to form the basis for the departmental culture.
7. Helping to communicate to staff and those outside the department just what that organization is all about.

WRITING A STATEMENT OF PURPOSE

The following list provides several helpful tips on writing and evaluating a purpose statement:

1. Make sure the mission statement of the department is directly related to the mission statement of the university.
2. Determine the specific portion of the university's mission statement the group is responsible to help achieve.
3. Prepare a rough draft of the mission statement that covers the purpose of the group and the major activities it performs.
4. With a working team a rough draft mission statement can be developed at an extended meeting. Using an outside facilitator who is familiar with communications techniques, group processes, and the concept of the mission statements is often helpful. The meeting can begin with each individual writing a version of the mission statement. When these drafts are all assembled, the group can review each one for clarity and understanding.
5. Consolidate those portions that are similar and negotiate within the group until there is general agreement on all points. The final result is the rough draft of the mission statement.
6. Submit the draft to the university president for review and input.
7. Finalize the statement.

An athletics department mission statement must be built around several points, such as:

1. The recruitment of student athletes who are capable of success in the academic program of the institution and the provision of academic support at a level that will effectively assist student athletes in reaching their potential.
2. Maintaining fiscal integrity by balancing budgets and carrying out sound business practices.
3. Fielding athletics teams that are successfully competitive with their peers.
4. Providing consistently outstanding customer service.
5. Careful compliance with institutional, conference, and NCAA rules.

SAMPLE MISSION STATEMENTS

At this point it might be helpful to examine sample mission statements prepared by three athletics departments. Note that these statements reflect the uniqueness of the departments in terms of their reason for being and also serve as guidelines for what the organizations should be doing. These statements were developed through a process involving many people and over a period of time that allowed reflection, deliberation, and input. Initial statements were revised a number of times to add specificity and clarity to the concepts and terms used to define purpose.

*   *   *

The University of Notre Dame has developed an excellent mission statement that represents its values. Portions of the Notre Dame Athletics Statement of Mission follow:

> The University of Notre Dame has embraced the philosophy that a well-rounded athletics program—including club, intramural, and intercollegiate competition—is an integral part of its educational mission. This philosophy also recognizes the importance of maintaining athletics programs in proper perspective in accord with the mission of the University as a Catholic institution of higher education. For this reason, Notre Dame is dedicated to the principle that the pursuit of excellence in intercollegiate athletics must be accomplished within the framework of an academic community committed to its educational objectives.
>
> *Academics:* Notre Dame is committed to being an environment of teaching and learning that fosters the development in its students of those disciplined habits of mind, body, and spirit that characterize educated, skilled, and free human beings. The University is committed to providing, on an equitable basis, ongoing opportunities that develop the moral, intellectual, and physical welfare of its students.
>
> *Student Life:* The student-athlete is first of all a student, who should experience the University of Notre Dame in the same way as the rest of the student body. Each student-athlete is held to the same standards of conduct as all other students.
>
> *Coaching Staff:* The University will strive to maintain a coaching staff of men and women who represent the best in athletics

instruction and who possess the ability to motivate and inspire the student-athletes for whom they are responsible. Coaches are primarily teachers. They share with members of the faculty and other university personnel the responsibility to educate, train, and assist in the formation of students entrusted to them. Coaches are expected to abide by the highest standards of personal conduct, and are expected to be role models for their student-athletes in how to pursue success with integrity.

Athletic Administration: Notre Dame will endeavor to maintain a high-quality, competitive athletics program consistent with its tradition and heritage. A full athletics program, consistent with the financial resources available, the athletics interests of the student body, and the overall academic mission and program of the University, will be provided for student-athletes. Club, intramural, and recreational athletics opportunities will be provided sufficient support so that all students may, if they desire, participate in some form of organized athletics activity.

Conclusion: In summary, as an institution, Notre Dame will pursue a standard of achievement in athletics consistent with its overall mission as a Catholic university. It will attempt to excel in every form of intercollegiate athletics without distorting its primary role as an educator and moral guide. Athletics programs are to be conducted in such a manner as to complement the goals of the commitment of the University to education, as well as the letter and spirit of the rules and regulations of the NCAA.

The University of Maryland athletics department has also integrated into its comprehensive statement of purpose an explicit statement of its "operational culture." This statement focuses on the issues of accountability, productivity, creativity, and a spirit of cooperation and teamwork—where employees view themselves as service centers to their internal and external customers.

Beyond a statement of purpose, it is often necessary for individual units within a department to develop their own guiding statements. For example:

1. The University of Tulsa Academic Support Unit for student athletes developed this mission statement: "The primary purpose of the program is to increase the graduation rates of student-athletes within the tenure of their athletic eligibility. This purpose is accomplished by improving the overall ability and increasing the desire of student-athletes to excel in the academic environment of the University of Tulsa. The program builds self-esteem and increases self-definition, self-responsibility, and self-motivation. It requires nothing less than full and active participation on the part of student athletes, which invariably increases their level of academic and social maturity, thus having a positive effect on the rate of graduation."

2. The mission of the University of Oklahoma Athletic Development Unit is, "(1) To provide monies and resources for the overall Athletic Department Plan; (2) To serve as one of the public relations arms of the athletic department; (3) To create a positive environment for our customers . . ."

EVALUATING A PURPOSE STATEMENT

The following list can be used as a guide to evaluate a statement of purpose. The goal is to devise a statement that authentically represents what the organization wants to be or should be to survive:

1. *Broadness of scope and continuity of application.* The statement should be broad enough to cover all significant areas of activity expected of the organization, without a specific termination period indicated.

2. *Functional commitment.* The nature of the works, tasks, or activities to be performed must be defined in terms that will clearly determine the validity of the group or organization.

3. *Resource commitment.* The statement should include a commitment to cost-effective utilization of available resources.

4. *Unique or distinctive nature of work.* Every unit in an organization should make some unique or at least distinctive contribution. If there are two or more peer units in an organization with identical missions statements, the risk of duplicated effort is obvious.

5. *Description of programs, events, and services to be offered.*
6. *Description of group or groups to be served.*
7. *Geographical area to be covered.*

Sometimes it is useful to use a series of questions to evaluate a purpose statement after it is written. A "no" answer to any of the questions means the statement needs to be reworded with more clarity in order to reflect the athletics department's basic reason for being. The following list of questions may be useful:

1. Does it contain all important commitments?
2. Does it clearly state the function?
3. Is there a clear determination of relationship to the rest of the organization?
4. Is it distinct from the mission statements of other groups in the organization?
5. Is it reasonably brief, to the point, and understandable?
6. Is it continuing in nature?
7. Does it state to whom the group is accountable?
8. Does it indicate the scope of service and reputation that the department wishes to establish—local, regional, national?
9. Does it address the important concept of service?

The purpose statement needs to answer the question of why the department is needed in the first place. It should discuss and define specifically what needs the department is meeting and the intended level of quality at which it aims to function.

SUMMARY

By verbalizing and putting in writing the vision and purpose of the athletics department, you are stating the unique reason why the department was brought into existence in this specific setting. This provides a sense of direction and focus for what you do. What you do is a function of who you are. The purpose statement worksheet which follows should provide the rationale (based on sound purpose) for the existence of the athletics program in your college.

PURPOSE STATEMENT WORKSHEET

1. Write a brief purpose statement for any three of the function areas of an athletics department (such as the compliance office, the academic support unit, the strength and conditioning areas, the sports medicine unit, the media relations office, or the business office):

    (a) First Area (Name):
       Purpose Statement:

    _____

    _____

    _____

    _____

    (b) Second Area (Name):
       Purpose Statement:

    _____

    _____

    _____

    _____

    (c) Third Area (Name):
       Purpose Statement:

    _____

    _____

    _____

    _____

2. Now, reflecting on the (overall) purpose of the athletics department as a whole, write a brief purpose statement for the department.

_____

_____

_____

_____

3. Evaluate the statements using the list of questions provided on p. 35.

_____

_____

_____

_____

4. Next, submit it to someone familiar with the department to evaluate and offer suggestions on improving the statement. In other words, does the statement say to others what you want it to say? List three or more individuals (e.g., the Faculty Athletics Representative, a member of the Athletic Council, an athletics department friend or booster who has a balanced view of its role within the institution, a selected student athlete, a parent of a student athlete, a member of the institution's administration, a member of the governing board or other appropriate individuals) who could offer insight and helpful responses. Below each person listed, indicate the reason(s) why you selected that person.

(a) Response/Input Resource Person #1 (Name and/or Title): Reasons Selected:

_____

_____

_____

_____

(b) Response/Input Resource Person #2 (Name and/or Title):
Reasons Selected:

_____

_____

_____

_____

(c) Response/Input Resource Person #3 (Name and/or Title):
Reasons Selected:

_____

_____

_____

_____

Chapter 4

Analysis and Assumptions

In this chapter, we will first discuss the absolutely essential need to assess the environment within which an athletics department operates, in order to understand the nature of external trends and influences. Next, we will address the important role of internal analysis of the department's operational culture, its focus or emphasis, the nature and scope of its resources, the level of its achievements (i.e., its past/traditions, its present financial conditions, competitiveness, graduation rates, etc.), and its self-image. It is critical that all attributes (whether strengths or weaknesses) of the organization be understood as well as the features of its external environment (consisting of opportunities and threats) in order to establish appropriate assumptions on which to develop plans. Consequently, this step is essential to the success of the strategic planning process.

EXTERNAL ANALYSIS: ATHLETICS IN THE MIDST OF RAPID CHANGE

It is vital for an athletics department to gauge the environment within which it operates. Indeed, this should be standard practice for all organizations. It is important to realize that anything that can happen probably will, and that there is no completely accurate way to predict what the future will bring. The only way we can manage change is to constantly monitor the environment within which we function. Examples for business might be the trends we see in gross national product, government control, regulation, the labor movement, interest rates, consumer preference, industry surveys, marketing research, Dow Jones stock averages, or recent commodity prices.

This environmental analysis stage is where we look at the past, identify current trends, and take the pulse of the environment in which the athletics department must survive and succeed. Remember, environmental analysis must not be confused with the process of making assumptions, which will be discussed later.

An environmental analysis for a department of athletics might include the following elements:

1. There are two professional sports franchises within a fifty-mile radius of the campus, with another professional team (a National Hockey League team) projected to be added to this sports market in the next twelve months.
2. These two franchises have significantly increased their marketing thrust throughout the past two years and have thus increased their market share of the sports ticket-buying public.
3. Media coverage and public interest is perceptibly shifting toward the professional sports teams in the region and away from collegiate athletics as a central point of interest.
4. In the past eighteen months, two of the seventeen corporate sponsors of the athletics program have discontinued their sponsorship and have become corporate sponsors of one of the two professional teams.
5. Court decisions establishing acceptable formulas for compliance with Title IX regulations have resulted in numerous financial challenges to the department.
6. The department's conference has realigned its revenue-sharing formula for member institutions in a way that will impact and challenge the department.
7. The proliferation and increased market penetration of televised collegiate football and basketball games has impacted the public's willingness to purchase tickets for and attend local collegiate games. In this local market, over 400 televised professional and NCAA football and basketball games were available via broadcast and cable television this year.
8. Current legal initiatives are underway to mandate financial subsidy for each scholarship athlete among the almost 600 student athletes on the athletics department's sports teams.

9. The institution's campus development program includes taking two of the department's six athletic fields for a building site and a parking garage during the next two years.
10. NCAA sanctions placed on the department will limit television and bowl appearances over the next twenty-four months.
11. The academic calendar of the university has been altered in a way that impacts the scheduling of athletics events, especially in the revenue sports.
12. The institution has raised the minimum GPA and entering standardized test scores required for regular admissions.
13. The institution has changed the number of academic "special admits" that are available to the department and its prospective student athletes.
14. There is a growing spectator interest in women's sports teams, with a potentially significant upside for ticket sales for the competitions of three of the women's teams.
15. The complex and increasingly difficult issues of sports gambling, aggressive sports agents, substance abuse, and similarly challenging trends are clearly beginning to impact this athletics program.
16. There is a growing impact of television on the scheduling of sports events in the revenue sports.
17. There has been significant economic upturn in our region of the state.

ASSESSING OPPORTUNITIES AND THREATS IN THE EXTERNAL ENVIRONMENT

One of the many possible external environmental factors can emerge or take precedence, sometimes with surprisingly short notice, thereby greatly changing the conditions under which the athletics department functions. The key is to constantly monitor and assess the external environment to best anticipate and plan for these possible exigencies. Indeed, opportunities and threats (or significant challenges) related to the external environment must be identified and carefully analyzed in order to determine what action (strategy) is appropriate to deal with them.

Further, opportunities will remain unrealized unless they are identified as such and analyzed as to their potential benefit. Likewise, recognizing threats (significant challenges to the viability of the department's strategies) and analyzing the possible ramifications of these trends or events help avoid many difficulties and crises. Some have referred to this as "what if" and "what then" analysis. In other words, asking the questions "What if this happens" and then "What do we do if this happens?" helps an athletics department deal with major events or trends that might be detrimental to the department.

This stage in the planning process does not merely involve gathering data related to external factors and getting it on paper. The external environment must be constantly monitored and the gathered information must be analyzed and used as an integral planning tool.

INTERNAL ANALYSIS

At the departmental level, internal analysis can include a complete study of the department's focus, management system, policies, outcomes, and other factors; as well as a review of the management system. A questionnaire/survey can give management information on the effectiveness of the system and can help reveal any major problems. It should address the planning environment, organizational structure, management philosophy and style, planning process, and other factors relating to the organization. The result is a thorough understanding of the planning system.

A method for auditing the planning system is also needed. The data collected in the audit can then be analyzed to determine strengths and weaknesses in the planning system. The most important arc then included in the strengths and weaknesses part of the planning process.

Many successful businesses are continually doing research to learn more about their customers. An athletics department should do this also. Information can be gathered on such factors as family size, marital status, age levels, where people work, people's needs, how long members have been associated with the athletics department, and where they live. Developing this kind of database allows the athletics department to plan much more effectively and also to better understand its customers and more effectively meet their needs.

It is important for the athletics department to build and maintain a thorough database. The more readily available and useful information on file is, the better opportunity that management has to make timely and sound business decisions. An old adage says, "your decisions are only as good as your information." The more you know about your finances, your outcomes over time in all areas of the department, and the people you serve, the better the department will understand itself as a part of its internal analysis.

For example, one athletics organization surveyed its customers and found (among many other factors) that 53 percent were under age thirty-five, 28 percent had been associated with the organization one year or less, 52 percent lived within ten miles of the organization venue, 31 percent were single, 8 percent were single parents, etc. This and other kinds of customer information can be quite useful in program design and in marketing.

ASSESSING STRENGTHS AND WEAKNESSES

After you have identified the purpose and considered the environment in which you operate, it is important to objectively assess the strengths and weaknesses of the department. Planners can learn this from the strategies of coaches. Coaches are constantly assessing the strengths and weaknesses of their team and their opponents. They try to identify and then maximize their strengths on game day and then improve their weaknesses in practice. Organizations have certain strengths that make them uniquely suited to carry out their tasks. Conversely, they have certain weaknesses that inhibit their abilities to fulfill their purposes. Among the numerous elements to be evaluated are human, financial, facilities, equipment, and natural resources.

It is fairly easy to identify the strengths in each of these areas. When you attempt to define weaknesses, it becomes a little more uncomfortable. Often, organizations must engage outside consultants to be able to candidly identify their limitations. But weaknesses and limitations must be recognized before you move on. All the evaluations listed in the environmental analysis can be separated into strengths and weaknesses.

Often athletics planning groups identify strengths first and write them so they can be analyzed openly and candidly, sometimes on a chalkboard in full view of the group. Through discussions, the group agrees on perhaps five major strengths. Then, each person writes two or three weaknesses of the organization that are added to the board to generate discussion. Only with a candid appraisal of strengths and weaknesses can realistic objectives be set.

MAKING ASSUMPTIONS

The next step is to make assumptions about spheres over which you have little or absolutely no control (e.g., the external environment). One good place to start is to extend some of the items studied in the external analysis.

Assumptions inherent in the field of athletics management might well include such statements as:

1. Television and radio programming costs will continue to increase dramatically, especially during prime time.
2. Tax issues will remain constant related to athletics donations, tickets, etc.
3. Title IX will remain a priority item in athletics.
4. The most successful coaches will remain with the athletics program, especially in the major revenue sports.

A list of certain assumptions that characterize the athletics department should be developed. Assumptions are those thoughts and ideas that we take for granted about ourselves, and other important factors. These assumptions are basic beginning points in a department's commitments and programming.

SUMMARY

This chapter emphasized the importance of coming to grips with the external and internal environments in which you must work to fulfill your mission. Minimizing weaknesses and capitalizing on strengths helps bolster the ability of an organization to operate in its external environment. Specifying the assumptions provides a basis for thoughtful consideration of the basic premises on which you operate. They should also cause you to ponder the "What if" and "What then" scenarios that help avoid disruptions in the organization's operations through contingency planning. The following "Analysis and Assumptions Worksheet" will aid you in applying these concepts.

ANALYSIS AND ASSUMPTIONS WORKSHEET

1. **List key environmental factors for your plan.**

   Institutional:
   1. _____
   2. _____
   3. _____
   4. _____

   Conference:
   1. _____
   2. _____
   3. _____
   4. _____

   Regional:
   1. _____
   2. _____
   3. _____
   4. _____

   Local:
   1. _____
   2. _____
   3. _____
   4. _____

   National (including federal issues, the NCAA, etc.):
   1. _____
   2. _____
   3. _____
   4. _____

Chapter 5

Establishing Objectives

In this chapter we discuss establishing objectives, the third step in the strategic planning process. After the purpose or mission of the athletics department has been defined, internal and external analysis completed, and assumptions made, then, and only then, can objectives be considered effectively.

You cannot achieve goals if you do not have any. This idea is so simple that many people overlook it. To accomplish anything, we must first purpose in our hearts to do it. We have to make up our minds. If we do not, we just waste our time and energy and find ourselves dissipating our resources, then looking back at the past, wondering where they went.

NATURE AND ROLE OF OBJECTIVES IN INTERCOLLEGIATE ATHLETICS

The terms key results, goals, and targets are often used synonymously when speaking of long- and short-term objectives. Whatever the term used, the idea is to focus on a specific set of target activities and outcomes to be accomplished. Think of the analogy of the archer used earlier. An Athletic Administrator wants the department aimed at the target just as an archer wants his arrow aimed at the bull's-eye. People get confused and disorganized if they do not know where they are going. The success or failure of an athletics program is often based on its ability to set specific and measurable goals, as well as on having tools with which to measure progress.

There are at least six reasons why athletics departments fail to set clear-cut objectives.

1. Sometimes Athletic Administrators wish to avoid the kind of accountability that is inherent in specific and measurable objectives.
2. Many projects seem destined to continue even when they no longer serve the department's reason for being or its mission.
3. Departments sometimes undertake activities for which money is available rather than because the activities are germane to its purpose.
4. Some Athletic Managers fear that hard-nosed evaluation may undermine the entitlements that former coaches, employees who are graduates of the institution, or former athletes at the institution, sometimes feel they have to be employed or continue their employment based on their perceived status.
5. The skills or interest needed to develop objectives and execute an effective strategic plan may not be present.
6. Athletic Administrators in many settings must spend an inordinate portion of their time in activities such as fund-raising and public relations. They must also frequently meet with university representatives, legislators, donors, conference and NCAA personnel, parents, representatives of the media, and others of their numerous publics. Therefore, they have not made time to lead in the establishment of a strategic planning process that includes relevant, clear, challenging, and measurable goals for the athletics program. An Athletic Director in such a setting in a major conference recently observed, privately, "The conference, institutional, NCAA, legal and media issues seemingly come at us in waves. So much so that clearly I do not have the time and energy remaining to give needed attention to the internal processes of goal-setting, outcomes evaluation and efficiency studies which I know would make us a better athletic department. That's just the way it is in this environment."

Objectives are clear, concise written statements outlining what is to be accomplished in key areas in a certain time period, in objective and *measurable* terms. Objectives can be classified as routine, problem solving, innovative, team, personal, and budget performance. Drucker states that "objectives are not fate; they are direction. They are not commands, but they are commitments. They do not determine the future, but they are the means by which the resources and energies of the operation can be mobilized for the making of the future" (Drucker, 1954, p. 102). Objectives can be set at upper organizational levels in areas such as growth, finances, physical resources, staff development, and attitudes. They are also needed in subunits, units, or divisions of an organization. Most important, all organizational objectives must be consistent. Thus, a unit's objectives should lead to accomplishing the overall departmental goals.

Objectives serve two fundamental purposes. First, they serve as a road map. Objectives are the results desired upon completion of the planning period. In the absence of objectives, no sense of direction can be attained in decision making. In planning, objectives answer one of the basic questions posed in the planning process: Where do we want to go? These objectives become the focal point for strategy decisions.

The second basic purpose served by objectives is in the evaluation of performance. The objectives in the strategic plan become the yardsticks used to evaluate performance. It is impossible to evaluate performance without some standard with which results can be compared. The objectives become the standards for evaluating performance because they are the statement of results desired by the planners.

Objectives are often considered the neglected area of management because in many situations there is a failure to set objectives, or the objectives that are set forth are unsound and therefore lose much of their effectiveness. In fact, one approach to management, called management by objectives (MBO), has emphasized the need for setting objectives as a basic managerial process (Migliore, 1983).

ALTERNATIVES TO MANAGING BY OBJECTIVES

One way to be convinced of the usefulness and power of managing by objectives is to consider some of the alternatives (Thompson and Strickland, 1986, p. 52):

Managing By Extrapolation (MBE). This approach relies on the principle "If it ain't broke, don't fix it." The basic idea is to keep on doing about the same things in about the same ways because what you are doing (1) works well enough and (2) has gotten you this far. The basic assumption is that, for whatever reason, "your act is together," so why be concerned about the establishment of goals and objectives?

Managing By Crisis (MBC). This approach to administration is based upon the concept that the strength of any really good manager is problem solving. Since there are plenty of crises around, "enough to keep everyone occupied," managers ought to focus their time and energy on solving the most pressing problems of today. MBC is, essentially, reactive rather than proactive, and the events that occur dictate management decisions.

Managing By Subjectives (MBS). The MBS approach occurs when no organization-wide consensus or clear-cut directives exist on which way to head and what to do. Each manager translates this to mean "do your best to accomplish what you think should be done." This is a "do your own thing the best way you know how" approach. This is also referred to as "the mystery approach." Managers are left on their own with no clear direction ever articulated by senior management.

Managing By Hope (MBH). In this approach, decisions are predicated on the hope that they will work out and that good times are just around the corner. It is based on the belief that if you try hard enough and long enough, then things are bound to get better. Poor performance is attributed to unexpected events and the fact that decisions always have uncertainties and surprises. Much time is therefore spent hoping and wishing things will get better.

All four of these approaches represent "muddling through." Absent is any effort to calculate what is needed to influence an organization's direction and what its activities should be to reach specific objectives. In contrast, managing by objectives is more likely to achieve targeted results and have a sense of direction.

CHARACTERISTICS OF GOOD OBJECTIVES

For objectives to serve as a means of providing direction and as a standard for evaluation, they must possess certain characteristics. The more of these attributes possessed by a given objective, the more likely it will achieve its basic purpose. Sound objectives should have the following characteristics:

1. *Objectives should be clear and concise.* There should not be any room for misunderstanding what results are sought in a given objective. The use of long statements with words or phrases that may be defined or interpreted in different ways by different people should be avoided.
2. *Objectives should be in written form.* This helps to provide effective communication and to discourage the altering of unwritten objectives over time. Everyone realizes that oral statements can be unintentionally altered as they are communicated. Written statements avoid this problem and permit ease of communication. Indeed, unwritten objectives tend to be altered to fit current circumstances.
3. *Objectives should name specific results in key areas.* The key areas in which objectives are needed will be identified later in this chapter. Specific desired results, such as "100,000 dollars in annual contributions" rather than a "high level of contributions" or "an acceptable level of contributions," should be used to avoid doubt about what result is sought.
4. *Objectives should be stated for a specific time period.* For example, objectives that set for a short run, more immediate time period such as six months to one year, must be accomplished as a prerequisite to longer-run objectives. The time period specified becomes a deadline for producing results and also sets up the final evaluation of the success of a strategy.
5. *Objectives should be stated in measurable terms.* Concepts that do not allow precise definition and qualification should be avoided. "Goodwill" is an example of a concept that is impor-

tant, but which in itself is difficult to define and measure. An objective related to goodwill that would be capable of quantification might be stated as follows: "To have at least 85 percent of our constituents rate our athletics department as one of integrity and competitive excellence, providing consistently outstanding customer service and academic outcomes." This is to be assessed by a survey of relevant constituents. Phrases such as "high attendance at athletics events" not only are not clear or specific, but cannot be measured. Does high mean first, second, or third in attendance? Is it a specific number, or a percentage? If the statement is quantified as "Increase attendance by 20 percent in two years" it can be objectively measured. The accomplishment or failure of such a stated objective can be readily evaluated.

6. *Objectives must be consistent with overall organization objectives and purpose.* This idea has been previously stated, but must be continually reemphasized because of the need for organizational unity.

7. *Objectives should be attainable, but of sufficient challenge to stimulate effort.* Two problems can be avoided if this characteristic is achieved. One is the avoidance of frustration produced by objectives that cannot be attained, or that cannot be attained within the specified time period. If an athletics program already has an unusually large attendance at a majority of its events, then the preference and likelihood of substantial increases in attendance are doubtful. The other problem is setting objectives that are so easy to attain that only minimum effort is needed. This results in an unrealistic performance evaluation and does not maximize the contribution of a given strategic plan.

One approach to writing objectives that contain these characteristics is to apply a set of criteria to each statement to increase the probability of good objectives. One such list follows:

1. *Relevance.* Are the objectives related to and supportive of the basic purpose of the athletics department?

2. *Practicality.* Do the objectives take into consideration obvious constraints?

3. *Challenge.* Do the objectives provide a challenge?
4. *Measurability.* Are the objectives capable of some form of quantification, if only on an order-of-magnitude basis?
5. *Schedule.* Are the objectives so constituted that they can be time phased and monitored at interim points to ensure progress toward their attainment?
6. *Balance.* Do the objectives provide for a proportional emphasis on all activities and keep the strengths and weaknesses of the organization in proper balance?

Objectives that meet such criteria are much more likely to serve their intended purpose. The resulting statements can then serve as the directing force in the development of strategy. Consider the following examples of poorly stated objectives:

* *Poor:* Our objective is to maximize attendance at home football games.

  Critique: How much is "maximum?" The statement is not subject to measurement. What criterion or yardstick will be used to determine if and when actual attendance is equal to the maximum? No target dates are specified.

  Better: Our objective is to achieve an attendance target average of 67,000 per game for home football games within three years.

* *Poor:* Our objective is to increase contributions to our department of athletics.

  Critique: How much? A one-dollar increase will meet that objective, but is that really the desired target?

  Better: Our objective for the next fiscal year is to increase private gifts to athletics from $5.7 million to $6.2 million.

* *Poor:* Our objective is to boost marketing/advertising expenditures by 15 percent.

  Critique: Marketing is an activity, not a result. The marketing objective should be stated in terms of what result the extra marketing activities are intended to produce.

Better: Our objective is to boost our ticket sales across all sports by 20 percent over the next two years, aided by a 15 percent increase in marketing expenditures.

- *Poor:* Our objective is to be the best athletics department in the conference.

Critique: Not specific enough; what measures of "best" are to be used? Attendance? Championships? Quality of customer service?

Better: We will strive to become the number-one athletics department in the conference in graduation rates, competitive success, and customer service within three years.

TYPES OF OBJECTIVES INCLUDED IN A STRATEGIC PLAN FOR ATHLETICS

Objectives can be set in areas such as attendance at athletics events, number of sports offered, level or degree of compliance with Federal Title IX requirements, fund-raising dollars for operational and/or capital needs, the level of competitive achievement in sports for which the conference and/or the NCAA conducts championship competitions, and any number of other "Key Result Areas" that are typical of most athletics programs. For example, "Key Result Areas" for setting objectives could include:

- Revenue by sport
- Championships
- Wins/losses
- Graduation rate
- Public attendance at games, by sport
- Budget
- Community service
- NCAA certification of the athletics department

Attendance Objectives

Attendance objectives are integral to athletics programs for several reasons:

1. The level of attendance is a tangible measure of the value that has been created for the fan or customers. It measures the value of your product to the target groups for whom the events are staged.
2. Higher attendance levels at revenue sports events have a desired effect on department revenues.
3. Well-attended events send a positive message to potential recruits and their parents who attend the events.
4. Large, enthusiastic audiences at events generate increased media attention, school spirit, competitive efforts, and a positive image of success for the department and the institution.

Attendance objectives can be stated numerically or as a percentage increase. If the objectives are stated in percentages, they also need to be converted to numbers for budgeting and estimating the audience size. Examples of attendance objectives are given in Exhibit 5.1. The way objectives are stated must reflect what the department can realistically expect to attain during a given plan. Also, the steps of setting objectives and developing strategy in preparing a marketing plan should be viewed as interactive. In setting objectives, we first state them in terms of what we want to accomplish, but as we develop the strategy we may discover that we cannot afford what we want. The available resources committed to a given program may not be sufficient to achieve a stated objective; and if the planning process is resource-controlled, the objectives must be altered. It must be remembered that objectives are not fate, but they are direction. They are not commands, but they become commitments. As a planner, you must not fall into the trap of thinking that once objectives are set they cannot be altered.

EXHIBIT 5.1. Examples of Attendance-Oriented Objectives

1. Achieve average attendance of 67,000 for home football games within three years.
2. Have 20 percent of the potential TV audience view our hosted conference baseball tournament championship game.

Each of the objectives in Exhibit 5.1 is clear, concise, quantifiable, and stated within a given time period. Only the second objective requires external data to evaluate whether it was accomplished, because total audience size would be required to compute the percentage.

Fund-Raising Objectives

Private gifts are a vital part of most athletics departments. They are the enabling resources that are needed, and indeed, required, in today's athletics environment. However, there is a more practical reason for including a specific statement about fund-raising: It forces the planner to estimate the resources needed to underwrite specific programs and operations. A statement of whether resources will be available cannot be made without at least some analysis of the cost of providing services for activities that must break even. For new activities, the expenditures and contributions associated with the activity should have been analyzed before the activity or program was launched. For existing programs, contributions can be analyzed to project continued levels of support. This information, combined with estimates of expenses involved in implementing the fund-raising strategy, provides a basis for statements of objectives about contributions.

Sample statements are shown in Exhibit 5.2 as illustrations of fund-raising objectives. Again, nebulous statements such as "acceptable fund-raising levels" or "reasonable contributions" should be avoided because of the possible variations in definition and the lack of quantifiability and therefore measurability. The objective of a percentage increase in contributions is the only one requiring additional information for its evaluation, because the amount of the

EXHIBIT 5.2. Examples of Fund-Raising Objectives

1. Produce net annual donations of $6.8 million within five years.
2. Generate a 20 percent increase in contributions within five years.
3. Produce contributions of $4.7 million for scholarship costs within three years.

total previous contribution would be required to determine whether this objective has been reached.

Keep in mind that the interactive processes of setting objectives and developing strategies must be used to set objectives that are realistic. The costs of many aspects of strategy cannot be estimated until a written statement of strategy is developed. If the strategy calls for a new program, for example, that strategy must be spelled out in detail before costs can be estimated.

Constituent Objectives

Constituent objectives may seem unusual to some, but their inclusion should be obvious. They serve as enabling objectives in the areas of:

- Academic and competitive outcomes produced by one of the most important constituent groups of any athletics program, that is, the student athletes.
- Attendance by fans at athletics events.
- Contributions by donors.
- Approval and acceptance of the activities of the department by the university community and various other publics. These constituent objectives also represent specific statements of constituent behaviors and attitudes that an athletics department would want its constituencies to have toward its programs and services.

Constituent objectives are especially important in providing direction to the development of the strategy section of the plan. As shown in Exhibit 5.3, they specify results desired of constituents in terms of behaviors and attitudes and should have the same characteristics as

EXHIBIT 5.3. Examples of Constituent Objectives

---

1. Create at least 60 percent attendance at home football games by the student body within three years.
2. Have at least 75 percent of our constituents rate the quality of our programs and services as "good" or higher in a survey of fans.

---

other objectives. They must be stated in objectively measurable terms and should be evaluated in relation to their accomplishment as a part of the monitoring and control system used in the plan.

USING ENVIRONMENTAL ANALYSIS DATA TO SET OBJECTIVES

The objectives of a given plan are based on the data provided in the analysis discussed earlier. In other words, good objectives are based on a careful analysis of the external and internal environment of the athletic department. A specific example of how data are used in setting objectives may help in understanding this point.

A large athletics program had a declining number of people attending women's basketball games. The department had an arena capacity of 4,500 for use by the women's basketball team (the men played in an arena which seated 14,500 and sold it out for most games). The environmental factors were, for the most part, favorable, with a large population base of males and females within easy driving distance of the university's women's basketball games and a very active female youth population who participated in youth, middle school, and high school athletics, including a large participation rate and support base for women's basketball at those levels.

The analysis identified possible market segments to be targeted for marketing the university's women's basketball program. An example of this type of analysis for one segment follows.

The estimated number of youth involved in sports programs (especially basketball) was secured from school and youth sports and associations' records. Next, potential interest in attending the university's games was assessed through a telephone survey of a sample of 150 youths who participate in sports. The resulting analysis is shown in Exhibit 5.4.

Objectives derived through such a process represent the realities of the environment and also the willingness and ability of the athletics department to commit itself to such objectives. This example should also reemphasize the logic in the strategic planning format. The analysis precedes the setting of objectives, because realistic objectives must be derived from the results of the meaningful analysis.

EXHIBIT 5.4. Potential for Attracting Youths to Women's Basketball Games

---

Population in metropolitan area = 750,000.
Number of youths in the area (10 to 18 years old) = 86,000.
Number of youths participating in sports teams at all levels = 13,500.
Percentage of youths in telephone survey who say they are interested in attending one or more of the university's women's basketball home games—15 percent (or a projected estimate of 2,000 potential fans from a cultivated base of 13,500 youth sports participants).

Objective: Attract an average of 600 youths per home game within three years, to be added to the average crowd of 1,800 who currently attend women's basketball games (other groups can also be identified, objectives set, and strategies designed to be reached in order to further enhance attendance).

PERFORMANCE CONTRACTS

Objectives can become the basis of a performance contract for staff members. As an example, note how the objectives for an associate director of athletics for development (fund-raising) can become a performance contract through the following process:

- Properly written objectives submitted to the director of athletics.
- Items discussed and negotiated with the director.
- Objectives resubmitted to the director.
- List approved by both parties.
- In some organizations, both parties sign an objectives sheet designating an agreement that these specific and measurable objectives will be achieved within a specified time frame.

PERIODIC REVIEW

One practical way to record, communicate, measure, and update objectives is through a "Performance Plan Book" or "Management Plan Book." All objectives for the organization should be in this book. (Note that it can be computer-based.) Objectives are to be reviewed each quarter and updated. The following are examples of how objectives can be listed, tracked, and presented for review. This process greatly reduces paperwork and provides a concise and convenient method for review. Examples are of overall department objectives that encourage a look into the future. They take into account key result areas.

OVERALL DEPARTMENTAL OBJECTIVES
(YEAR 1 TO YEAR 3)

STAFF	Year 1	Year 2	Year 3
Athletic Director			
Associate ADs			
Assistant ADs			
Unit Heads			
Others			

ATTENDANCE	Year 1	Year 2	Year 3
Revenue sports			
Nonrevenue (Olympic) sports			

MEMBERSHIP IN THE BOOSTER CLUB	Year 1	Year 2	Year 3
Total private gifts to athletics			
Raw numbers of members			
Rate of growth, percentage			
Average annual donation per member			
Other issues			

FACILITIES AND MAJOR EQUIPMENT	Year 1	Year 2	Year 3
Facilities construction			
Facilities improvement			
Added major equipment			
Safety and security incidents			

ACADEMIC OUTCOMES	Year 1	Year 2	Year 3
Dropout rates			
Transfer rates			
Graduation rates			

Returning athlete Academic
  Assistance Program participation
  rates
Other

PROGRAMS	Year 1	Year 2	Year 3

Academic, counseling, and career
  assistance
Character awareness and development
  activities
Sports programs offered
Title IX compliance program
Customer service enhancement
  initiatives
Others

PEOPLE/TRAINING MORALE/ DEVELOPMENT	Year 1	Year 2	Year 3

Quality of the workplace program
Training and development
  opportunities
Attitude and morale surveys
Employee feedback program
Special assistance programs

PUBLIC RESPONSIBILITY	Year 1	Year 2	Year 3

Use facilities for civic and other groups
Social and educational activities by staff
  and student-athletes
Educational opportunities for student-
  athletes related to public conduct,
  alcohol, treatment of the opposite sex,
  gambling, etc.
Events opened at a discount or free to
  disadvantaged individuals and groups
Others

FINANCIAL	Year 1	Year 2	Year 3

Budget issues
Revenue enhancement issues
Cost containment issues
Financial integrity issues
(See also booster club issues)

REVIEW SHEET
MANAGEMENT PLAN, YEAR 1

ROUTINE

Set aside $225,000 each year for four years to serve as a special contingency reserve for athletics operations. On target.	25% completed

PROBLEM SOLVING

Budgeting system that allows closer monthly tracking of expenditures (raw dollars and percentage of each sport budget expended) for each of the 26 sports in the athletics department. Complete by end of the current fiscal year.	90% completed

INNOVATIVE

Devise a more effective plan for assessing the quality of customer service in every relevant area of the department during the current year.	70% completed

PERSONAL

Read the book *Strategic Planning for Collegiate Athletics* and attend at least one relevant management seminar during the current year.	50% completed

BUDGET PERFORMANCE

Operate within the $28 million athletics budget throughout Fiscal Year 1.	On target

ATHLETIC ADMINISTRATOR'S OBJECTIVES, YEAR 1

ROUTINE

Conduct at least one plenary staff meeting each month.

Review each employee's objectives and accomplishments each six-month period (each direct-report employee).

Attend the regular meetings of the booster club board.

Prepare a standard agenda for my regular biweekly meeting with my supervisor.

Prepare a topical agenda for distribution to the Faculty Athletics Council in connection with my monthly report to that group.

PROBLEM SOLVING

Develop cost-containment guidelines for the department as a whole.

Set up a Cost-Containment Committee to review the guidelines, revise as needed, and to set up a program for implementation of the guidelines across the department. The committee should be made up of administrators, coaches, staff, and two student-athletes.

Develop a plan to enhance the quality of the workplace for all employees, using a survey to assess employee morale and preferences regarding work environment.

Sponsor a quarterly luncheon for all employees to provide a time of fellowship, reporting on our successes and challenges, to solicit feedback from employees, and to openly discuss the theme for the year: "Commitment to Excellence and the Will to Win."

Develop guidelines regarding the continuing eligibility of student-athletes who are charged with or convicted of a misdemeanor or felony offense while enrolled and participating as a student athlete in the university.

INNOVATIVE

Devise an enhanced system of screening prospective student-athletes with regard to their probable success or failure in the academic program of the university.

Develop a method to provide all appropriate employees interim feedback on their budget performance.

PERSONAL

Improve my relationship with selected boosters who are potentially important to the athletics department, but who have been alienated by practices of previous administrators.

Exercise with other staff in department facilities at the times when they are most frequently present.

Upgrade management skills by attending a technology-related management seminar.

TEAM

Work with my direct reports on improving ways we can communicate more efficiently on routine and urgent operational issues.

Meet regularly with the administrator who is responsible for fund-raising, along with the elected layman president of the booster club, to enhance the coordination and direction of our current efforts to generate additional private support of athletics.

BUDGET

Operate within the established annual expense budget.

Retire 20 percent of the debt on our most recent capital project.

Prepare a proposal to implement zero-based budgeting for the department.

SUMMARY

Setting objectives is another major part of the strategic planning process in athletics. The necessity for objectives as well as their needed characteristics was presented here to lay the groundwork for identifying basic types of objectives, such as attendance, fund-raising, and constituents. The objectives provided as examples in this chapter can be used both as a source of direction and to evaluate the strategies developed for your plan. The following "Objectives Worksheet" will aid you in applying the concepts in this chapter to your athletics department or similar organization.

OBJECTIVES WORKSHEET

Answer These Questions First

What do your objectives need to relate to attendance, fund-raising, constituents, or all three? What are your other key result areas?

_____

_____

_____

_____

What needs to happen for your department or unit to be successful? In other words, how many people need to attend/watch, join, contribute, volunteer, graduate, win, etc.?

_____

_____

_____

_____

When do you want this to happen? By what specific date?

_____

_____

_____

_____

Now Write Your Objectives

Draw upon the information in your answers to the above three questions and other resources in order to write statements of your objectives.

Objective 1:

_____

_____

_____

_____

Objective 2:

_____

_____

_____

_____

Objective 3:

_____

_____

_____

_____

Now test each statement using the criteria given in this chapter. Is each statement relevant to the basic purpose of your organization? Is each statement practical? Does each statement provide a challenge? Is each statement put in objectively measurable terms? Do you have a specific date for completion? Does each statement contribute to a balance of activities in line with your department's strengths and weaknesses?

Chapter 6

Developing Strategy and Operational Plans

After developing a set of objectives for the time period covered by the strategic plan, you must formulate the strategy needed to accomplish *each* of those objectives. You will first design an overall strategy. Then you must plan the operating details of that strategy (as it relates to the total efforts of the athletic department) in order to guide those efforts with specific strategies designed to achieve each written objective.

STRATEGY CONCEPTS

The word "strategy" has been used in a number of ways over the years, especially in the context of business. Often, it is confused with the terms "objectives," "policies," "procedures," and "tactics." Strategy may be defined as the course of action taken by an organization to achieve its objectives. It is the catalyst or dynamic element of managing that enables a company, an athletics department, or any organization to accomplish its objectives.

Strategy development is both a science and an art and is a product of both logic and creativity. The scientific aspect deals with assembling and allocating the resources necessary to achieve an organization's objectives with emphasis on opportunities, costs, and time. The art of strategy is mainly concerned with the utilization of resources, including motivation of the people, sensitivity to the priorities of your environment, and ability to adapt to changing conditions.

ALTERNATIVE STRATEGIES

Alternative strategies should be evaluated by management before committing to a specific course of action outlined in the strategic plan. Thus, strategy is the link between objectives and results.

There are two basic strategies that an athletics department can use to accomplish its objectives: a differentiated strategy and a focused strategy. The chosen strategy must of course be an outgrowth of the organization's basic purpose.

Differentiated Strategy

A differentiated strategy is a strategy that entails developing services that are aimed at meeting a broad spectrum of needs. It is the strategy used by most organizations that develop a whole gamut of programs. Research has shown that this is the best strategy for new or underperforming organizations that are attempting to attract broad interest and support. This kind of organization will typically offer a wide range of services and programs aimed at a broad spectrum of target groups in order to attempt to build an extensive and often diverse base of participation and support. Each program and service to be provided will need to develop specific strategies for the objectives it has established.

By using a differentiated strategy, an organization thus targets a broad segment of markets, with programs and services marketed to appropriate groups and subgroups.

Focus Strategy

A focus strategy is more likely to be used by an organization because it involves concentrating on the needs of a specific group or on a specific type of activity.

The main advantages of this strategy are: (1) it capitalizes on the distinctive competencies of the people involved, and (2) it concentrates on doing a focused or limited number of things well. These advantages can also create a knowledge base of how to carry out focused types of activities effectively, as well as improved efficiency in performing those activities or programs.

FACTORS INFLUENCING THE STRATEGY SELECTED

At least four factors influence the choice of a strategy selected by an athletics department: (1) the organization's resources, (2) the distinctive competencies of leaders and staff, (3) stage in the organization's life cycle, and (4) strategies used by other organizations. There is no one best strategy that will always prove successful. Instead, the strategy that is chosen must be the one that is best for the specific athletics department, given the nature of these four factors. Resources, for example, can limit the organization to a focused strategy. The organization may even be an innovator in terms of ideas but not have the financial, communication, or personnel resources to offer other services.

As was emphasized in Chapter 2, the organization strategy must be derived from the organizational purpose and objectives. If the organizational purpose is focused on serving needs of diverse groups, then the strategy used must be one that is compatible. In other words, what an organization *does* must be a function of what it *is*.

The distinctive competencies of the organization have a direct bearing on the strategy selected. These distinctive competencies are the basis of doing things well. Smart, well-managed organizations always build upon their strengths.

The organization's life-cycle stage is an additional factor influencing strategy selection. For example, an organization may begin with a focus strategy but add programs over time that serve more varied needs. Repositioning the organization through introducing new programs or serving new markets would be a pivotal point of the strategy.

The strategy selected must be given sufficient time to be implemented and affect groups served, but an obviously ineffective strategy should be changed. This concept should be understood without mention, but resistance to change is a common phenomenon in many organizations.

OPERATIONAL PLANS

After all the steps have been taken and a strategy has been developed to meet your objectives and goals, it is time to create an operational or action plan. The operational plan is the "action" or "doing" stage. Here you hire, develop, build, advertise, and so on. How many times has a group of people planned something, become enthusiastic about it, and then nothing happened? This is usually because group leaders did not complete an operational or action plan to implement their strategy.

Operational plans must be developed in all the areas that are used to support the overall strategy. These include sports programs, communication, finance, and staffing. Each of these more detailed plans is designed to spell out what needs to happen in a given area of the athletics department in order to implement the strategic plan.

The production plan identifies exactly what programs and services will be provided to a specific group and the exact nature of those services.

The communication plan is used to communicate to the constituency and staff the nature and purpose of the activity or program, its location, and time frame. This plan also needs to be well thought out and carefully analyzed to avoid miscommunication.

The communication strategy involves three key elements: informing, persuading, and reminding.

Informing

Informing involves providing information to individuals and groups about the organization. Specific elements of the plan call for:

1. Use of video cassette presentations
2. Newsletters and pamphlets
3. Personal speaking appearances by leaders
4. Hosting luncheons/dinners sponsored by the organization and its supporters
5. On-site visits by individuals/groups to the organization

Persuading

Persuading involves presenting and selling the purpose and programs.

1. Provide compelling information and inspiration to target groups.
2. Share opportunities to provide volunteer and/or financial support for the program.

Reminding

Reminding is continuing to provide information to people already familiar with the program so they will be constantly aware of the work and needs of the department.

1. Send letters/newsletters and other materials regularly.
2. Provide opportunities for team members to write fans and supporters on a periodic basis.
3. Develop a complete file of individuals and groups by name for future mailings.

In the staffing plan you must identify who will carry out the activities involved. Will it be department staff or volunteers? If paid staff are to be used, will they be full-time or part-time? Of course, if volunteers are to be used they must be recruited, trained, and supervised.

Finances must also be planned, usually in the form of a financial budget. The budget is the means to execute the plan. If the financial means to support the plan are not available, you must adjust the objectives. There is a constant interplay between the budget and the plan. Many people do not understand the budgeting process. The budget is a tool; too often, however, the budget becomes the "tail wagging the dog." "We budgeted it so we had better spend"; "We had better add a little to this year's budget"; or "That has never been in the budget, so it cannot be something we should be doing," are statements that reflect this misunderstanding. Budget money must be tied directly to performance, and performance is measured against objectives. Key results and objectives in an athletics department are prioritized and then money and resources are allocated.

An example of this budget and plan interplay came out of a meeting at a large organization. Most of their resources for the next two years would have to go into finishing current building programs. Only enough money was available to maintain the status quo of parts of the organization that were deemed appropriate for growth and expansion. That does not mean the expansion is not important—it is—but the timing for expansion and growth for the organization cannot come until the other projects are completed.

The action plan for a large department with many different types of programs and services is depicted in Exhibits 6.1 and 6.2 (only a

EXHIBIT 6.1. Action Plan: Academic Support Unit (Student-Athlete Graduation Rates)

OBJECTIVE:

To achieve a 78 percent graduation rate in the next five years (Year 1-Year 5)

    Year 1: 67 percent graduation rate

    Year 2: 70 percent graduation rate

    Year 3: 74 percent graduation rate

    Year 4: 76 percent graduation rate

    Year 5: 78 percent graduation rate

STRATEGIES:

A. We plan to increase year by year, as better prepared student-athletes are recruited and as we improve our academic-status monitoring system.

B. We plan to add three professionals (two part-time and one full-time) to the tutorial staff each year for the next four years.

ACTION PLAN	PERSON RESPONSIBLE	START DATE	DATE COMPLETED
1. The Assistant Athletic Director for Academic Services/Career Development is hiring and training one administrative professional this year and is also hiring and monitoring the activities and effectiveness of three additional tutors this academic year.			
2. Others			

---

limited number of action steps are provided). The operational or action plan in this example is related directly to the strategy to be used and the objectives to be accomplished in a step-by-step fashion. This forces the planner to align objectives, strategies, and action plans.

EXHIBIT 6.2. Action Plan: The Development (Fund-Raising) Unit

---

OBJECTIVE:

To increase private support of athletics to $7.4 million in five years

    Year 1: $5.2 million

    Year 2: $5.6 million

    Year 3: $6.1 million

    Year 4: $6.8 million

    Year 5: $7.4 million

STRATEGIES:

A. Develop a competent volunteer (peer-group) fund-raising cadre to work with the four staff professionals.

B. Develop a refined computer database of potential impact donors.

C. Develop a plan to strengthen the historically weak alumni-athletics financial support behaviors.

D. Initiate more cooperative efforts between athletics and the institutional development office of the university.

E. Hire an additional fund-raising administrator/professional.

ACTION PLAN	PERSON RESPONSIBLE	START DATE	DATE COMPLETED
1. Add staff to the donor tracking system staff and train these persons by the unit head during the current year.			
2. Direct mail the full alumni list with news of the department and outlining our financial needs once each year for the next three years, to be carried out by the fund-raising unit.			
3. Others			

Notice that the action plan format takes one objective out of the five-year strategic plan and isolates it for further study and analysis. In this case it provides an example or two of the targets at which this department is aiming with its Academic Support Unit and its Development Unit.

Never go into action until the target is clear and understood by everyone. It is important that all those who execute these plans be integrally involved in the planning. That is the key to enthusiasm and support by the staff.

With targets/objectives/goals in mind, various strategies are agreed upon. *They are listed immediately under the objectives.* Next, all the actions that must take place are listed. Also note that at the top of each section is a row to write who is in charge, date started, and date completed. This document becomes not only a guide to action but a timeline for starting and completing plans.

The person or persons responsible and the expected date of completion must be agreed upon. Every person involved gets a copy of the plan with his or her areas of responsibility clearly indicated. Often one person can coordinate a multitude of projects and programs because there is a clear record of what is to be done. As each action or task is completed, the person responsible submits a complete report. With this approach, the coordinator knows the status of the plan and knows what is going on continuously.

The action plan is periodically updated so that everyone sees the progress. After people become accustomed to using the action plan format, they discipline themselves. They do not want others to observe that they are falling behind. This is a great time-saving and coordinating tool. In Appendix B we present a sample strategic plan in an abbreviated/descriptive form to illustrate the development of strategy and action to accomplish a mission. Appendix C provides a detailed sample of an athletics strategic plan.

SUMMARY

A well-conceived plan developed by everyone succeeds. How often do we see athletics programs trying to do everything at once? The word "strategic" in the title of this book implies thinking, developing, and specifying priorities and order. All this can happen if the action plan coordinates and supports the overall plan, and also *relates to each specific objective* in the strategic plan. The following "Strategy Development Worksheet" is provided to help you apply the concepts discussed in this chapter to your organization.

STRATEGY DEVELOPMENT WORKSHEET

Answer These Questions First

1. What are the distinctive strengths and competencies of your athletics department? What do you do well?

_____

_____

_____

_____

2. What market segment or segments should you select to match your organization's programs and resources to (and constituents' perceived needs in those segments)?

_____

_____

_____

_____

3. Do you have the skills/resources to pursue several segments or should you concentrate on one segment? Is that segment large enough to sustain your desired growth?

_____

_____

_____

_____

Now Develop Your Positioning Statement

1. Distinctive Competencies

_____

_____

_____

_____

2. Segments Sought

_____

_____

_____

_____

3. Programs and Services Offered

_____

_____

_____

_____

4. Promotion Orientation

_____

_____

_____

_____

5. Contribution Levels

_____

_____

_____

_____

6. Growth Orientation

_____

_____

_____

_____

Chapter 7

Evaluation and Control Procedures: Monitoring, Feedback, and Reward

The evaluation and control (monitoring) stage of the strategic planning process is like consulting a road map while on a journey. The process includes identifying your destination (objective), determining the best route to your destination (strategy), and then departing for your trip (implementation of your strategy). During the journey, you look for highway signs (feedback) to tell you if you are on the way to your objective (Dowling and Miller, 1987). Signs along the way quickly reveal if you have made a wrong turn and you can alter your course to get back on the correct road. When you reach your destination, you decide on a new route (strategy) to get you somewhere else.

Imagine what would happen if there were no road signs during your trip to let you know if you were on the right road. It might be too late or too costly to continue the trip by the time you realized you were traveling in the wrong direction. Yet, many organizations are involved in a similar situation, failing to analyze results to determine if objectives are being accomplished.

Failure to establish procedures to evaluate and control the strategic plan can lead to less than optimal performance. Many organizations fail to understand the importance of establishing procedures to appraise and control the planning process. In this chapter we review the need for evaluation and control, what is to be controlled, and some control procedures. Evaluation and control should be a natural follow-through in developing a plan. No plan should be considered complete until controls are identified and the procedures for recording and transmitting control information to administrators of the plan are established.

INTEGRATION OF PLANNING AND CONTROL

Control should be an integral part of the planning process. Planning is a process that includes establishing a system for feedback of results. This feedback reflects the organization's performance in reaching its objectives through implementation of the strategic plan. The relationship between planning and control is depicted in Exhibit 7.1.

The strategic planning process results in a strategic plan. This plan is implemented (activities are performed in the manner described in the plan) and results are produced. These results include such things as attendance; contributions; and accompanying constituent attitudes, preferences, and behaviors. Information on these results and other key result areas is given to administrators, who compare the results with objectives to evaluate performance. In this performance evaluation they identify the areas where decisions

EXHIBIT 7.1. Planning and Control Process

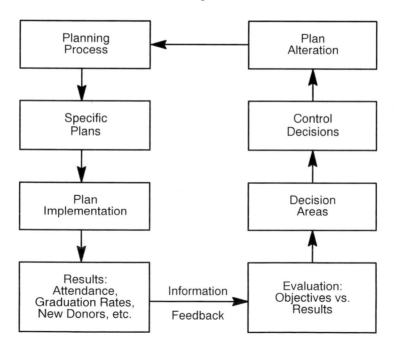

must be made to adjust activities, people, or finances. Through this decision making the administrators control the plan by altering it to accomplish stated objectives, and a new cycle begins. The information flows are the key to a good control system.

The last stage of the strategic planning process, then, is to appraise the organization and each of its entities, to determine if all objectives of the strategic plan have been met.

- Have the measurable objectives and goals been accomplished?
- How far did actual performance miss the mark? Did the attainment of the objectives and goals support the overall purpose?
- Has the environment changed enough to now change the objectives and goals?
- Have additional weaknesses been revealed that will influence changing the objectives of the organization?
- Have additional strengths been added or your position improved sufficiently to influence the changing of your objectives?
- Has the organization provided its constituencies (internal and external) with rewards, both extrinsic and intrinsic?
- Is there a feedback system to help constituencies satisfy their needs?

As stated previously, the strategic plan is supported by operational plans. If each operational plan is controlled properly, the strategic plan itself is more likely to be efficiently controlled. The administrator cannot afford to wait for the time period of a plan to pass before control information is available. The information must be available within a time frame that is long enough to allow results to accrue, but short enough to allow actions to align results with objectives. Although some types of organizations may find weekly or bimonthly results necessary, most organizations can adequately control operations with monthly or quarterly reports. Cumulative monthly or quarterly reports become annual reports, which, in turn, become the feedback needed to monitor and control the plan. Deciding what information is provided to which administrators in what time periods is the essence of a control and monitoring system.

PERFORMANCE EVALUATION AND CONTROL

Performance should be evaluated in many areas, to provide a complete analysis of what results are and what caused them. Key control areas are those such as event attendance, private gifts in support of the athletics program, constituent attitudes (fans, donors, alumni, etc.) and graduation rates. The following is a discussion of three of these areas.

Attendance Monitoring and Control

Attendance or audience control data are provided from an analysis of attendance at games for individual sports teams. Attendance can be evaluated on a team-by-team basis by developing performance reports as shown in Exhibit 7.2. When such a format is used, the attendance objectives stated in the plan are broken down on an annual basis and become the standard against which actual attendance results are compared. Number and percentage variations are calculated, because in some instances a small percentage results in a large number variation.

A performance index can be calculated by dividing actual attendance by the attendance objective. Index numbers near 1.00 indicate that expected and actual performance are about equal. Numbers larger than 1.00 indicate above-expected performance and numbers below 1.00 reveal below-expected performance. Index numbers are especially useful when a large number of sports are involved, because they enable administrators to identify those programs or sports that need immediate attention (see Exhibit 7.2).

EXHIBIT 7.2. Attendance and Performance Report (By Sports Team)

Sports Team	Attendance Objective (avg)	Actual Attendance	Variation	% Performance Variation	Index
A	10,000	9,000	1,000	−10.0	.90
B	950	1,020	+70	+7.4	1.07
C	1,200	920	−280	−23.0	.77
D	2,000	2,030	+30	+1.5	1.02

Contribution/Cost Controls

Several tools are available for establishing cost control procedures, including budgets, expense ratios, and activity-costs analysis. Budgets are a common tool used by many organizations for both planning and control. The budget is often established by using historical percentages of various expenses as a percentage of revenues. Thus, once the total level of expected contributions is established, expense items can be budgeted as a percentage of total revenues. If zero-based budgeting is used, the objectives to be accomplished must be specified and the expenditures necessary to accomplish these objectives estimated. The estimates are the budgeted expenses for the time period.

Contributions are monitored and controlled by tracking gifts on a monthly or quarterly basis. While many athletics programs have an annual drive for pledges, others are continually seeking contributions from potential donors. A prerequisite to controlling/establishing needed contribution levels is an annual projection of operating expenses. This projection, broken down on a quarterly or monthly basis, becomes the standard from which deviations are analyzed. For example, a small department with a projected budget of $2 million for the next fiscal year would expect to average about $500,000 per quarter, or about $167,668 per month in total income, with a carefully weighted percentage of that coming from contributions.

If there were large variations related to certain times of the year, even the variations can be analyzed to determine the proportion of the budgeted amount given per month.

The same type of analysis used to monitor and control attendance (see Exhibit 7.2) can be used to analyze data on contributions. This type of analysis should be performed on a timely basis.

Once the budget is established, expense variance analysis by line item or expenditure category is used to control costs. A typical procedure is to prepare monthly or quarterly budget reports showing the amount budgeted for the time period and the dollar percentage variation from the budgeted amount, if any exists. Expenditure patterns that vary from the budgeted amounts are then analyzed to determine why the variations occurred. This way, the budgetary issues and functions as related to achieving the strategic plan are adequately monitored and thus serve to help meet the objectives of the plan.

Constituent Feedback

The final area of performance evaluation that we will discuss is constituents and involves analysis of awareness; knowledge; and attitudes and behaviors of fans, participants, and donors. Every organization should want its constituents to become aware of programs, services, or personnel; possess certain knowledge; and exhibit certain attitudes and behaviors. If these are specified in the objectives statement, they are the standards to which current constituent data are compared.

Data on constituents must be collected on a regular basis. There are many ways to collect data, but surveys are commonly used. Constituent data are especially valuable if collected over a long period of time, because awareness levels, satisfaction, attitudes, and behaviors can be analyzed to reveal trends and areas for further investigation.

The University of Maryland has a comprehensive and continuous calling program carried out by a staff member who spends about 25 percent of her work schedule in this effort. Season ticket holders, donors at various levels, and other fans are called throughout the year to thank them for their support and also to ask them to assess the programs and services of the athletics department and provide specific feedback regarding what they would like to see changed or improved. This has provided not only valuable feedback, but has also generated enormous goodwill among hundreds of individuals whom the department has called in the first eighteen months of this program. As part of *almost every interview* most produce an expression of surprise and gratitude that their satisfaction and input is important enough to the department that they would be called to be thanked for their support and asked for their input. As one representative fan and donor said, "I have not ever before had any business or group call me to thank me for my patronage and support or to ask my opinion on things. This is a first and I greatly appreciate it." The feedback received through this program has been extremely helpful to management, especially in the area of planning.

ESTABLISHING PROCEDURES

None of the performance evaluation data described are going to be available unless they are requested and funds are made available to finance these surveys and other methods. Thus, data collecting and reporting procedures must be set up by the administrators who are going to use the control data in decision making.

The procedures will usually change over time, as new types of analysis or report times are found to be better than others. The most important requirement is that the data meet the needs of administrators in taking corrective actions in order to control activities. With the expanded availability and use of computers by organizations, these functions can be much more effectively carried out within those organizations.

STAFF PERFORMANCE EVALUATION GUIDELINES

Keep these summary guidelines in mind when establishing an effective system for the specific area of employee performance evaluation:

1. Performance evaluation should include self-evaluation.
2. Performance evaluation should be intended to aid in the development of dedicated, performing, growing individuals.
3. Evaluation is in part subjective.
4. "No evaluation" is not an option.
5. When an evaluation process is perceived as relevant, fair, and effective, people will tend to use it responsibly. When it is not, people will still do something, but they may not feel that it is a compelling responsibility.
6. Performance evaluation is a formal process.

Individual performance assessment is a vital part of the evaluation and control step in intercollegiate athletics programs. This is true in part because *increasingly* these departments are being viewed by their institutions as accountable, along with other departments within the institution, to carry out equitable, systematic, and fair personnel hiring, development, and assessment procedures. And rightfully so.

Rewards, reprimands, or remedial/developmental measures must be related to the personal achievement or lack of achievement of agreed-upon objectives in the strategic plan. This creates a work environment where people know what to do and where rewards are tied to performance.

Reality reminds us each day that *employees are unfinished products.* As employees they require assessment and evaluation against measurable objectives, but some will need assistance and development, with the goal of becoming increasingly effective in their work. For this reason, progressive athletics departments across the United States are using comprehensive, systematic, developmental employee assessment programs.

One such program of employee evaluation is that which is used at the University of Maryland, where the work of every staff member (from the grounds keepers to coaches to the Athletic Director) is regularly and thoroughly evaluated using a written, comprehensive, standard format. Integral to this multistep process at Maryland is the concept that employees *can* and in most cases *will* develop and become more effective in direct relationship to: (a) their understanding of the achievement objectives that are expected of them, (b) the degree to which they are held accountable for performance, (c) their opportunities to receive feedback, support, and suggestions for improvement, and (d) their systematic and timely opportunities for learning and professional development under an enlightened and enabling supervisor.

The results of a stringent performance review and development program can be positive for the athletics department as a whole.

In Appendix D you will find sample performance review and development forms that are used as a part of the University of Maryland PRD Employee Evaluation Program. The emphasis is equally on *development,* along with the concept of *performance review.* They typically want to know how to do a better job within the department and therefore become more effective employees. This is especially true when they buy into the mission and purpose of the athletics department and understand the achievement objectives that are expected of them.

It is in the appraisal and control stage that organizations really begin to see the benefits of the strategic concepts outlined in this book. When people at all levels know the progress being made toward fulfilling the overall plan, it creates a sense of pride, accomplishment, and excitement. Strategic planning will not work well without a review of performance—both individual personnel performance and organizational performance related to the objectives in the athletics department's strategic plan.

REWARDING EXCEPTIONAL ACHIEVEMENT

In addition to evaluating performance, a system needs to be developed to reward those who are accomplishing their objectives, especially exceptional performers. This creates a vital link between performance and the reward system. Failure to reward exceptional performance may lead to demotivating employees rather than motivating them. Therefore, rewarding performance becomes very important. A system of bonuses might be used to pay for performance. Recent court rulings on equal pay make this an even more important topic for the future. One university just recently approved bonuses equal to one month's pay for the football and baseball coaching staffs. A number of collegiate football coaches are paid in excess of $50,000 each for postseason bowl appearances. As has been commonly observed, "You get what you reward." A bonus pool for everyone involved in the athletics department may be appropriate. For example, graduation rates, class attendance, competitive excellence, staff and student-athlete involvement in the community could all be tied to a reward system. Another interesting twist could be for the coach's bonus to be based on a minimum GPA, class attendance and graduation rate.

SUMMARY

No planning process should be considered complete until evaluation and control procedures have been established. Performance evaluation is vital for control decisions. Information tells an administrator what has happened and serves as the basis for any actions needed to control the activities of the organization toward predetermined objectives. Without such information, it is impossible to manage with a sense of clarity about what is actually happening in the organization and likewise to develop and effectively carry out a comprehensive strategic plan.

The important management practice of a thorough evaluation of outcomes (the determination of the level at which every objective of the department has been achieved) and the feedback that this process naturally provides is crucial to proper assessment of the success of a strategic plan. It is also integral to sound management practice in any enterprise.

Finally, the level at which each unit within the department and each individual employee achieve in reaching their objectives serves as the basis for rewards and recognition of these units and individual employees. This kind of merit-based reward system is the preeminent and most effective way to enhance performance toward meeting the strategic goals and objectives of the department. The following "Evaluation and Control Worksheet" will aid you in applying these concepts to your organization and its individual units.

EVALUATION AND CONTROL WORKSHEET

Answer the Following Questions

1. What kinds of information do you need to evaluate a program's or service's success?

_____

_____

_____

_____

2. Who should receive and review this information?

_____

_____

_____

_____

3. What time periods do you want to use to analyze the data? Weekly? Monthly? Quarterly? Annually?

_____

_____

_____

_____

4. What record keeping system is needed in order to make sure the information you want is recorded for the time periods you specified in Question 3?

_____

_____

_____

_____

Now Set Up Your Control Procedures

1. Specify the areas to be controlled:

    A. _____

    B. _____

    C. _____

    D. _____

2. Specify the format of the data for each area. (Is it to be numbers by period or by program? Do you want numbers and percentage variations?)

    A. _____

    B. _____

    C. _____

    D. _____

3. Specify how the data are to be collected, who is to collect and analyze the data, and who is to receive the results of the analysis.

    A. How will the data be collected?

    _____

    B. Who is responsible for collecting and analyzing the data?

    _____

    C. Who is to receive which type of analysis?

Administrators	Types of Analysis
1. _____	1. _____
2. _____	2. _____
3. _____	3. _____
4. _____	4. _____

Chapter 8

Raising Your Sights and Sharpening Your Tools Through the Use of a Planning Audit

The value of strategic planning in managing any enterprise cannot be overestimated. The multistep process of strategic planning that has been discussed in this book is a dynamic and effective management initiative. It means finding successful responses to a changing environment.

The heart of the planning process is setting specific, measurable, and attainable objectives for every unit within the department and for the department as a whole. This is to be followed by the development of appropriate strategies or steps needed for the achievement of each of these objectives. This process will almost always raise the sights of the department to achieve more challenging and worthy goals and objectives. It will also challenge and sharpen the human, financial, and procedural skills toward becoming a highly achieving organization. This happens when strategic planning is understood, embraced, and put into effect.

Effective strategic planning will turn around the very mentality of an athletics department and positively change its culture. It will create direction, cohesion, accountability, and improved outcomes. It is a powerful tool. It will alter the dynamics of the workplace. It will move an organization beyond coercion to cooperation and trust—to a shared vision and goals. It will achieve empowerment from the inside out (Migliore, Yow, and Bowden, 1998).

Planning will prepare an athletics department for change, even make it comfortable with change and adaptive behaviors. If an athletics department (or any organization) is not prepared for the change, it will be engulfed by it. If an organization is prepared for change it will be propelled forward by it. The intense competition for the entertainment dollar in our economy and the complex nature of growth in our business require a fleet-footed, responsive athletics organization—one which anticipates change well, one which continuously improves customer service to both internal and external customers, and one that skillfully builds on its strengths as an organization.

Effective strategic planning will raise an organization's sights and sharpen its tools in order to achieve at that higher level. Success begins with a plan. The future belongs to good planners. Planning is a process, a process that can be studied and improved. Improvements are centered on decisions concerning who will participate in the planning process and how the process will actually be executed.

This chapter focuses on how the planning process can be improved within an organization. The planning audit is described as a basic framework for analyzing the planning process and identifying specific actions to improve it. Improvements in the process result in better analysis, more realistic objectives, better strategies, and more appropriate control mechanisms.

THE PLANNING AUDIT

The concept of a planning audit was derived from accounting, where audits have traditionally been used as a procedure for internal financial control. The term can be defined in a number of ways: from simply a systematic and thorough examination of an organization situation to a *comprehensive, systematic, independent,* and *periodic* examination of the environment objectives, strategies, and activities with a view to determining problem areas and opportunities, and recommending a plan of action to improve performance. But, in essence, a *planning audit* is a critical, unbiased review of the philosophies, personnel, organization, purpose, objectives, procedures, and results associated with some activity. It is a review of everything associated with the planning process within an organization.

Audits are appropriate for virtually any type of organization— new to old, small to large, healthy or ailing, engaged in service, or physical products. The need for a planning audit may stem from a number of reasons; changes in target markets, in competitors, in internal capabilities, or in the economic environment. Consequently, an audit may have many purposes:

- It appraises the total operation.
- It centers on the evaluation of objectives and policies and the assumptions that underlie them.
- It aims for prognosis as well as diagnosis.
- It searches for opportunities and means for exploiting them as well as for weaknesses and means for their elimination.
- It practices preventive as well as curative administrative practices.

The audit process can be lengthy and complex. A great deal of prior planning and preparation are necessary. Ultimately, it involves (1) deciding who will do the audit; (2) agreeing on its objectives, scope, and breadth; (3) identifying sources of data; and (4) deciding on the format used to present its results.

AUDIT PERSONNEL

Basically the choice is between internal and external auditors. Internal auditors have the advantage of working relationships and familiarity with the organization's operating environment. If the audit is not a self-audit but is done by higher-level executives or an auditing staff, this approach can be less time-consuming and perhaps less costly. However, one basic assumption must be made for the full benefits of the audit to be realized when organization personnel are used: the internal auditors are not myopic in their knowledge of planning procedures. That is, they must have a good understanding of how planning should take place in any organization and not just in their particular organization. Unless the analysts possess the depth and breadth of knowledge needed in strategic planning, many of their judgments will be naive. It is not just an understanding of planning that is needed, but an understanding of strategic planning.

External auditors can provide some of the breadth of knowledge needed if their experience is broad-based. Consulting firms specializing in strategic planning may bring a perspective to the planning process that could not otherwise be obtained, especially for organizations with inbred executives. The major disadvantage of using external auditors is the time needed for them to gain an understanding of the organization's approach to planning and the qualifications and training of the people involved in the planning process. A long-term relationship with the same consulting group would help alleviate this shortcoming.

OBJECTIVE, SCOPE, AND BREADTH OF AUDIT

Audits should begin with a meeting between the organization officer(s) and the planning auditor(s) to work out an agreement on the objectives, coverage, depth, data sources, report format, and the time period for the audit. A detailed plan as to who is to be interviewed, the questions to be asked, the time and place of contact, and so on, is carefully prepared so that auditing time and cost are kept to a minimum. The cardinal rule in auditing is: don't rely solely on the organization's executives for data and opinion. Fans, alumni, and other outside groups must be interviewed. Many organizations do not really know how their constituents see them, nor do they fully understand constituents' needs.

The audit can be most effective when its philosophy is built on three attributes: comprehensive, systematic, and periodic. An audit should not be considered comprehensive unless all aspects of planning are analyzed. A revenue audit or promotional audit by itself provides depth but is not comprehensive enough to evaluate relationships among personnel, organization, and procedures. The audit must be comprehensive to be effective.

A systematic audit is one that follows logical, predetermined steps. An outline to such an approach is provided in the worksheet at the end of this chapter. The areas covered (based upon the major components of the strategic plan) and the types of questions asked provide the basis for systematically analyzing an organization.

This systematic approach should uncover a great deal of data about the planning process within an organization. Continually asking "why?" about procedures, decisions, and controls is the key to uncovering who did what with what efficiency and provides input for answering, "Are we doing the right things?"

The audit should be undertaken with sufficient periodicity to avoid crisis circumstances. Many organizations do not audit their managerial activities until a crisis has arisen, but in many cases a crisis can be avoided by an audit. Few strategic planning processes are so successful that yearly or second- or third-year audits should not be used.

AUDIT DATA AND REPORTING FORMAT

The data for the audit must be provided through source documents (attendance reports, contribution reports, budgets, or schedules) and interviews with personnel involved in planning. Top management must ensure that auditors have complete cooperation from these personnel and access to any information needed to complete the audit, especially when external auditors are used. Failure to provide access to the same data available to the planners is sure to lead to a superficial audit. Again, it is important to ensure that auditors have access to all constituent groups relevant to the situation. Failure to do so can result in an incomplete and misleading audit report.

Most companies assign one high-level executive as the key person for the external auditor to work through. Information requests routed through that executive carry authority by "virtue of office."

A variety of reporting formats is possible, but one of the most appropriate is a finding—a written report of recommendations. In such a report, the auditors' findings are written out for each area of study in the audit and a specific recommendation for improvement is stated for each finding. Thus the reporting format is action-oriented, and specific actions can be evaluated for improving the planning process.

INCREASING THE LEVEL OF SOPHISTICATION IN PLANNING

As the strategic planning process is used, audited, and restructured, it becomes possible to raise its level of sophistication. For example, once a database for attendance analysis or revenue fore-casting is established, other factors can be added or simulation models or input-output models can be developed. Online data re-trieval for control, as well as other improvements, can be made available for managers in companies with data processing equip-ment.

The important point to remember is that the level of sophistica-tion of the managers and planners should determine the level of sophistication used in planning. More training for current managers or hiring new managers with higher levels of skills permits move-ment of the planning process to more complex approaches.

SUMMARY

The final aspect of strategic planning, discussed in this chapter, is the planning audit. The audit is designed to improve the planning process within an organization and can increase the level of plan-ning sophistication. The strategic planning process can then be studied and improved through the analysis undertaken in the plan-ning audit. The following "Planning and Management Systems Au-dit Worksheet" will help you begin.

PLANNING AND MANAGEMENT SYSTEMS AUDIT WORKSHEET

I. Purpose
   A. Is it written?

   B. Does it define boundaries within which your athletics department operates?

   C. Does it define the needs that the department is attempting to meet? What are those needs?

      1. Student-athletes:

      2. College or university:

      3. Alumni:

      4. Fans and boosters:

      5. General public:

      6. Coaches and other employees:

      7. Others:

   D. Does it define the market that the department is reaching? Describe it.

E. What is its scope of outreach?

F. Has there been input from a wide range of personnel?

G. Does it include the concept of service as a part of this purpose or mission statement?

II. Environment Analysis
  A. Have you included all appropriate national trends that affect the department?

  B. Have you included state and local trends that affect the department?

  C. Have you identified trends unique to your department?
    1. Alumni base?

    2. Historical and emerging financial support?

    3. Average attendance at sports events?

  D. Have you included your most significant competitors?
    1. Which are growing?

    2. Which are declining?

    3. What are the successful ones doing?

III. Strengths and Weaknesses (Included for Each Area)
   A. People

   B. Facilities

   C. Financial

   D. Competitive advantage

   E. Image

   F. Others

IV. Functional Analysis
   A. Financial analysis
      1. What is your current financial situation?

         a. Do you have regular financial statements prepared?

      2. What tools would be beneficial in analysis?

         a. Do you have pro forma statements for profit centers such as the sportswear shop, licensing agreements, ticket sales, fund-raising, and others?

         b. Do you have a cash budget?

         c. Do you have a capital budget?

         d. Has a ratio analysis been prepared?

         e. Do you understand the time value of money?

         f. Do you understand and use break-even analysis?

      3. Have you analyzed current financial policies?

         a. Do you have cash policies?

       b. How are accounts receivable analyzed?

       c. How are accounts payable analyzed?

       d. Do you control inventory levels?

    4. Do you have a viable debt retirement plan?

    5. Do you periodically carry out a unit-by-unit and sport-by-sport cost-benefit analysis?

    6. Do you have effective cost-containment measures in place?

    7. What is a synopsis of your current financial situation?

B. Accounting analysis
    1. Analysis of current accounting policies
       a. Depreciation procedures?

       b. Tax considerations?

       c. Decentralized/centralized operations?

       d. Responsibility accounting?

    2. Tools beneficial in analysis
       a. Have you established short- and long-range budgets?

       b. Do you perform variance analysis?

       c. What costing methods are used?

       d. Do you perform contribution margin analysis?

    3. Are there adequate controls, especially of cash at events?

    4. What is your synopsis of the current accounting situation?

C. Market analysis
  1. Have you established marketing policies? What you will and will not do?

    a. Have you identified your consumers?

    b. Who are your competitors?

    c. Product: type of product, type of demand, market position?

    d. Distribution and location of facilities?

    e. Pricing and revenues?

    f. What promotion (advertising and selling) activities are you using?

  2. What is your synopsis of the current marketing situation?

D. Management analysis
  1. Do you have a planning system? How does it work?

  2. Are people and resources properly assigned?

  3. Is control centralized or decentralized?

  4. What staff needs do you have?

  5. Are controls in evidence? What are they?

  6. Is there a motivation or morale problem?

  7. Is strategy defined? What is the current strategy?

  8. How efficient are operations?

9. Is there a thorough and effective system for the evaluation of members of the management team? Are promotions, raises, and remedial action tied to their evaluations?

10. What is your synopsis of the current management situation?

V. Other Selected Areas of Analysis
   A. Computer systems
      1. Do you have a viable computer system in place?

      2. In what areas will it be used?
         a. Season ticket holder lists
         b. Mailings
         c. Financial systems
         d. Information systems
         e. Inventory control
         f. Fund-raising
         g. Payroll
         h. Other

   B. Legal analysis—Do you know the laws affecting your athletics department?

   C. Insurance: buildings, player injury or death liability, automobile liability, and related issues?

VI. Objectives
   A. Are the objectives in key result areas?

   B. Are the objectives specific, measurable, and for a set time frame with responsible individuals indicated?

   C. Are there intermediate and long-term objectives?

VII. Strategies—Do you have appropriate strategies for the achievement of each objective? Explain.

VIII. Competitive Analysis
    A. Is there a system to evaluate the specific competitive level of each sport in the department on a continuing basis?

    B. Is it designed for the conference and national levels?

Appendix A

Outline of a Strategic Plan

STRATEGIC PLANNING AND MANAGEMENT WORKSHEET

I. Purpose

What is the department's reason for being or its mission? Role of the athletics department with regard to the mission of the institution. Customers served. Needs met in the marketplace. Scope of the endeavor (nation-wide, regional, area):

II. Environmental Analysis

    A.

    B.

    C.

    D.

    E.

    F.

III. Strengths and Weaknesses

    A. Human

    B. Facilities/equipment

    C. Financial

    D. Competitive advantages/disadvantages

    E. Institutional issues (reputation, location, etc.)

    F. Other

IV. Assumptions

    A.

        1.

        2.

        3.

    B.

        1.

        2.

        3.

C.

    1.

    2.

    3.

V. Objectives and Goals (Desired Results, Outcomes, and Achievements)

A. Specific and measurable objectives in each key result area of the department, including a timeframe/target date for each.

B. Others

VI. Strategies (Two to Three for Each Objective)

A.

    1.

    2.

    3.

B.

    1.

    2.

    3.

C.

    1.

    2.

    3.

VII. Operational Plans and Controls

A.

B.

C.

VIII. Performance Appraisal/Rewards

A.

B.

C.

Appendix B

Summary Strategic Plan

STATEMENT OF PURPOSE

It is the purpose of Collegiate University Department of Athletics to provide a sound, competitive, intercollegiate athletics program that (1) represents the University in an impeccable manner and (2) provides student athletes the opportunity to develop physically, mentally, ethically, and socially. In doing so, the athletics program will provide:

a. *Coaching* of the finest quality, which keeps in balanced perspective the issues of competitive achievement and student athletes' development and well-being.

b. *Facilities* that provide excellent venues for safe and high-caliber competition.

c. *Academic assistance* that includes guidance and counseling, tutorial assistance, and all other appropriate academic services needed to enhance the academic success of the student-athlete—with a student-athlete's graduation being a preeminent goal.

d. *Customer service* that is consistently excellent in every area of the department—the ticket office; the cleanliness, maintenance, and safety of the physical facilities; game management; parent relations; alumni relations; donor benefits and services; media relations; and all other dimensions of the department.

e. *Other operations and initiatives* that build and maintain an intercollegiate athletics program of integrity and competitive excellence.

The athletics department will function within the overall mission of the university and shall conduct itself at all times in a manner that will enhance the educational experience of the student-athlete and contribute to the positive image of the institution.

ENVIRONMENTAL ANALYSIS

The department is committed to continuously monitoring and analyzing the environment in which it functions. In doing so it will understand the trends and issues of the environment that affect its present operations and outcomes and also understand the future conditions with which it must deal as an organization. It will monitor such issues as the following, in designing and executing its strategic plan:

a. Economic issues that relate to the economies of the institution, the area, state, and region in which the program functions. The economic conditions naturally have a significant effect on donor behaviors, and ticket-buying levels, and should be researched accordingly.

b. Demographic issues related to the population it serves and its target markets.

c. Conference issues such as revenue sharing trends, conference realignment, etc.

d. Federal issues (such as the interpretation of compliance with Title IX), present conditions, future trends.

e. NCAA and institutional issues and rules that could influence how the department functions and how it uses its resources.

f. Conditions of its own institutional setting such as admissions requirements, tuition increases, graduation requirements, and others.

g. The potential for proliferation of professional sports franchises in the area and state.

h. Other external environment factors.

In addition to *external* environmental factors to be explored as part of strategic planning, the department must also take a careful look at *internal* factors (present and future) such as changes in leadership, loss of successful coaches, aging of facilities, projected major equipment needs, and others.

A few examples of these environmental analyses follow:

a. Over a three year period, beginning in the 2000-2001 academic year, the university plans to raise its admission standard on the SAT by twenty-eight points and will not provide the athletics program with additional "special admits" for talented student-athletes.

b. The safety issues of our football stadium will require an expenditure of $2.5 million over a five-year period beginning this spring.

c. There appears to be financial backing in the city to bring an NBA franchise to the area within six years.

d. Current court interpretations of Federal Title IX will require $1 million in new facilities (office space, practice, and competition sites) and a $650,000 increase in the department's operating budget over the next three years.

e. The conference revenue-sharing formula will be altered for football and basketball in a manner that will reduce revenue to the department by approximately $68,000 per year, effective next year.

f. The NCAA share of postseason tournament revenues distributed to participating conferences (and subsequently to the institutions in our conference) might be reduced by 5 percent to 15 percent for the next five years, to allow the NCAA to pay the $80 million in damages (plus court costs and attorney fees of another $15 million) that were assessed against it on behalf of "limited earnings" assistant men's basketball coaches in their class action suit.

g. The present relative competitive strength of our athletics program will be maintained with regard to the sports teams of the other athletics programs in our conference, especially in the revenue sports.

In addition to an analysis of the internal and external factors, the department should also complete a thorough, candid analysis of its own strengths and weaknesses as a department and then integrate this information meaningfully into its strategic plan. Consider such areas as financial, organizational, human resources, market position, image, facilities, attendance levels, success or lack thereof in conference athletics competition, and Sears Cup standing (national competitive ranking across all sports).

ASSUMPTIONS

No long-range plan will be successful if the assumptions on which it is based are not clearly stated. Thus, in the case of the athletics program of Collegiate University, a number of major assumptions can be identified. These might be:

a. The present competitive strength of the sports offered will continue to maintain a place in the top half of the conference. Therefore most sports (particularly the revenue sports) will continue to experience their excellent level of attendance and revenues.

b. The revenue stream from private gifts to athletics will increase over the five year plan period at about 8 percent per year.
c. The conference will maintain its revenue sharing formula throughout the plan period, except as cited in b above.
d. The athletics "special admits" program will be maintained by the institution at its present level.
e. There will be no major changes in the present leadership of the department during the plan period.

OBJECTIVES

In this area of the strategic plan very specific, achievable, and measurable objectives are set for every area or unit within athletics, and for the department as a whole, for each year within the scope of the long-term strategic plan.

a. The athletics department (fund-raising) unit will increase its revenues by 25 percent during the five year term of the strategic plan.
b. The department will come into compliance with Federal Title IX guidelines within three years.
c. The department will move from the current #37 ranking in the Sears Cup competition to #25 or higher during the term of the strategic plan.
d. The student-athlete graduation rate will rise to equal or surpass that of the general student body during the term of this plan.

STRATEGIES

Specific enabling strategies should be written and placed under each objective. These are the steps that will be necessary (the specific work that must be carried out) to achieve each of the written objectives, along with who is responsible for doing each step and the desired time frame (or target date) for completing the step or strategy. A few samples of strategies (matched to above objectives) are as follows:

a. Objective A
   1. The fund-raising unit will develop a comprehensive grassroots campaign within the booster group to increase the membership in that group by 25 percent and increase scholarship support revenue by 20 percent. This will include peer group recruitment

and will be supported by extensive training and promotional materials provided by the staff.

2. An additional full-time major gifts fund-raiser will be hired and support personnel hired and trained.
3. Donor benefits will be carefully reviewed and increased at all donor levels to create additional customer value for membership and donations.

b. Objective B

1. The department will construct women's soccer and softball facilities.
2. Head coaches will be hired at least ten months prior to the start of competition.

c. Objective C

1. Recruiting budgets will be increased to match or surpass the average of a representative sampling of athletics programs presently ranked in the Top 25.
2. Coaches' contracts will include bonus payments for appearance in the NCAA tournament and thus earning Sears Cup points.

These strategies should also contain target dates and indicate the individuals responsible for the completion of each. The operational plan, or who is to do what and when, is built upon the objectives and their strategies for accomplishment.

EVALUATION, CONTROL, AND REWARD SYSTEM

As a part of the strategic plan, the department will set up a system by which the progress in achieving each objective by its target date is carefully monitored and feedback provided to appropriate persons. This is a prescribed, formal, and continuous process.

Quarterly, the head of each unit will review with each responsible employee the progress that has been made toward meeting the objectives within the unit, while the senior staff will meet quarterly with unit heads to review their progress and to analyze the progress toward meeting the department-wide objectives.

Updated, written summaries will be prepared as a result of these quarterly review/assessment meetings and made available to everyone involved in executing elements of the strategic plan. Employee evaluations, semiannual and annual, will be at least partially based on the individual's performance in effectively and efficiently executing the strategies needed to meet the objectives for which he or she is responsible.

Merit awards and other recognition will be provided to those performing at a high level. Likewise, those employees who have not demonstrated the commitment and work habits to achieve their objectives will be remedially addressed. In some cases where it has become clear that the objectives were not realistic, some adjustments may be in order.

At the end of the strategic plan time frame (usually a five year period), a comprehensive postprocess review is carried out by the department and a new planning process occurs for the next strategic plan period.

Note:

A detailed strategic plan for an average size NCAA Division I institution (sixteen to eighteen sports) will typically run approximately twenty-five to thirty-five pages. The previous brief summary/sample is presented simply to get you started in developing your strategic planning process and preparing your strategic plan document.

Appendix C

Detailed Strategic Plan

METRO UNIVERSITY
ATHLETICS DEPARTMENT
STRATEGIC PLANNING DOCUMENT
February (Year 0)
John Doe, Athletic Director

I. MISSION STATEMENT

Metro University is committed to developing a strong tradition of excellence in intercollegiate athletics. The Department of Athletics strives to instill in its student-athletes an appreciation for hard work and pride in accomplishment. It is believed these attributes will be utilized throughout the student-athlete's life.

II. ENVIRONMENTAL FACTORS

Listed below are key opportunities and threats for each of the following environmental sectors:

A. External Environment Analysis
  1. GOVERNMENT—NCAA Rules, Title IX
     a. Opportunities
        (1) Limit on scholarship, coaches—level playing field
        (2) Threat of Title IX not as great for us
     b. Threats
        (1) Student-athlete right to work
        (2) Title IX—financial limitations

2. ECONOMY—Marketing
   a. Opportunities
      (1) Local economy growing
      (2) Untapped community resources
      (3) Merchandising, group sales, promotions
   b. Threats
      (1) Limited entertainment funds
      (2) Other sporting events in local area

3. TECHNOLOGY
   a. Opportunities
      (1) Use technology to better evaluate athletic performance
      (2) Entertainment at events
      (3) Promote events and ticket sales
   b. Threats
      (1) Costs of equipment and personnel
      (2) TV, etc., may limit attendance
      (3) Technology may not be readily available

4. SOCIAL TRENDS
   a. Opportunities
      (1) Family fun entertainment
      (2) Affordable entertainment
   b. Threats
      (1) Competition from other entertainment sources
      (2) Athletics not as popular as TV, video games, and alternative sports

5. STUDENTS
   a. Opportunities
      (1) Greater student involvement
      (2) Diverse entertainment to market to student body
      (3) Use partial scholarship giveaways to increase involvement
   b. Threats
      (1) Conflicting meetings and apathy
      (2) Entrance requirements for student-athletes
      (3) Funding for student-athletes' summer jobs
      (4) Older-age students

6. FUNDING SOURCES/SPONSORSHIP
   a. Opportunities
      (1) Golden Badge Club

       (2) Corporations and foundations
       (3) Tickets, merchandise
    b. Threats
       (1) University image
       (2) Limited sponsorship funds
       (3) Competition for dollars

7. COMPETING EDUCATIONAL INSTITUTIONS
    a. Opportunities
       (1) Expanded recruiting base in conference cities
       (2) Expanded marketing opportunities in conference cities
    b. Threats
       (1) Nearby NCAA Division I universities
       (2) Other conference schools
       (3) Non-NCAA Division I universities and junior colleges

8. CONCLUSIONS FROM EXTERNAL ANALYSIS
    a. International/national trends that affect the university and the athletic department are:
       (1) Stronger and more competition in recruiting
       (2) Stronger and more competition in scheduling
       (3) More jobs for student athletes and athletics department personnel under new NCAA legislation
    b. Several local trends that affect the university and the athletics department are:
       (1) Stronger and more competition for attendance and funding of athletics programs
       (2) Growing local economy
       (3) Improving image of the university
    c. Trends unique to the university and the athletics department are:
       (1) Untapped funding sources in merchandising, group sales, and fundraising
       (2) Untapped attendance sources
    d. Our most important competitors are:
       (1) Nearby NCAA Division I universities with:
          (a) Local media coverage—brings more attention to athletics
          (b) More money in bigger conferences with more personnel
       (1) Some of the conference schools that are declining:
       (2) The successful ones are growing because:
          (a) Winning against bigger foes

(b) Recruiting better athletes

(c) Bigger sales forces

B. Internal Operations Analysis

Listed below are the key strengths and weaknesses for each of the following operational sectors of the university and the athletics department:

1. MANAGEMENT AND PLANNING SYSTEMS
    a. Strengths
        (1) Competent energetic personnel
        (2) Efficient operations for given resources
        (3) Good communication
    b. Weaknesses
        (1) Lack of management experience
        (2) Lack of firm plans and goals
        (3) additional staff needed in marketing and compliance, volleyball, computers, secretaries
        (4) Restrictive office space
        (5) University financial condition hinders our ability to get the best price for needed equipment, supplies, and services
        (6) Absence of needed personnel prevents ability to generate additional revenue from ticket sales and merchandise sales

2. FINANCIAL RESOURCES
    a. Strengths
        (1) Athletics department financial statements are prepared and reviewed regularly
        (2) Adequate resources are available for competition at current level
    b. Weaknesses
        (1) Funds are needed for additional personnel, recruiting, equipment, travel, and salaries
        (2) Payments and allocations need to be reported to athletics department more quickly
        (3) Limited number of alumni

3. MARKETING RESOURCES
    a. Strengths
        (1) Excellent department head—energetic
        (2) Better ideas and products than competitors
        (3) Great ticket prices and packages
    b. Weaknesses
        (1) Need to continue to rebuild image in community

       (2) Need to complete detailed written marketing plan

       (3) Need to further identify ticket buyers and funding sponsors

       (4) Need stronger student, faculty, alumni, and community support

       (5) Need greater demand for tickets and sponsorships

       (6) Need more personnel and advertising budget

   4. OPERATIONS OR SERVICES RESOURCES

     a. Strengths

       (1) Excellent athletics facilities

       (2) Ample size, great design

       (3) Excellent support from administration

     b. Weaknesses

       (1) Need some renovations and new facilities

       (2) Need some new equipment

       (3) Need more office space

       (4) Some conflicts with use of coliseum

III. ASSUMPTIONS

The following are the major assumptions upon which the athletics department has based its strategic plan:

1. Athletics department budgets will increase 3 percent to 5 percent per year
2. NCAA scholarship limitations and budget requirements will remain the same
3. Remain a member of our conference
4. Title IX will remain in effect
5. Athletic programs will remain competitive
6. University image in the community will continue to improve
7. Athletics programs will continue to receive full support of the University administration
8. Local economy will not regress
9. Student support will continue to improve

IV. AREAS, OBJECTIVES, AND ACTION PLANS

The following are Areas/Objectives and Action Plans for the athletics department for the next five years.

AREAS/OBJECTIVES FOR THE NEXT FIVE YEARS

AREAS/OBJECTIVES	Year 1	Year 2	Year 3	Year 4	Year 5
I. Academics					
A. GPA	2.65	2.70	2.75	2.80	2.85
B. Graduation rate (percentage of those who declare majors)	35	38	41	44	50
C. Expansion of Academic Learning Center					
1. Full-time counselors	0	0	1	1	2
2. Additional computers	4	2	2	2	2
3. Increase funding for additional resources by 10 percent each year	0	1,000	1,500	2,000	2,500
4. Life Skills/Community Service Program	1	2	3	3	3
II. Compliance					
A. Increase percentage of minority student-athletes	30%	32%	34%	35%	35%
B. Increase number of female student-athletes	42%	45%	48%	51%	54%
C. Increase funding for women's athletics	44K	88K	132K	176K	220K
D. Increase number of minority and female staff members	0	1	2	3	3
E. Add Senior Women's Administrator	0	1	1	1	1
III. Marketing					
A. Season ticket sales					
1. Men's and women's basketball	1,300	1,400	1,500	1,600	1,700
2. Baseball	200	225	250	275	300
3. Volleyball	50	75	100	125	150
4. Soccer	100	125	150	200	250
B. Group sales					
1. Men's and women's basketball	5,000	5,500	6,000	6,500	7,000
2. Baseball	200	250	300	350	400
3. Volleyball	50	100	150	200	250
4. Soccer	200	250	300	350	400

AREAS/OBJECTIVES	Year 1	Year 2	Year 3	Year 4	Year 5
C. Ticket revenue					
1. New season tickets	$17,250	$15,550	$17,050	$18,600	$20,300
2. Group sales	$12,950	$14,350	$15,750	$17,150	$18,550
3. Game day sales	$18,000	$19,000	$20,000	$21,000	$22,000
4. Total	$48,200	$48,900	$52,800	$56,750	$60,850
D. Attendance (per game)					
1. Men's and women's basketball					
a. Overall	5,000	5,250	5,500	5,750	6,000
b. University students, faculty, and staff	1,500	1,600	1,700	1,800	1,900
2. Baseball					
a. Overall	350	400	450	500	550
b. University students, faculty, and staff	50	75	100	125	150
3. Volleyball					
a. Overall	250	300	350	375	400
b. University students, faculty, and staff	200	225	250	275	300
4. Soccer					
a. Overall	300	350	400	450	300
b. University students, faculty, and staff	150	175	200	225	250
E. Sponsorship sales (cash and trade)					
1. Men's and women's basketball	40,000	43,800	44,500	46,000	47,500
2. Baseball	1,600	2,100	2,300	2,600	31,000
3. Volleyball	800	850	980	1,000	1,500
4. Soccer	750	800	900	975	1,050
F. Merchandising (% increase/sales)	10,000	20,000	30,000	40,000	50,000
G. Golden Badge Club development	75,000	100,000	125,000	150,000	175,000
H. Capital campaign	200,000	210,000	215,000	N/A	N/A
I. Additional staff	1	2	1	0	1
J. Broadcast affiliates	10	12	15	19	23

AREAS/OBJECTIVES	Year 1	Year 2	Year 3	Year 4	Year 5
IV. Competition					
A. Tier I sports (men's basketball, women's basketball, volleyball, baseball)					
1. Winning percentage	60	62.5	65	67.5	67.5
2. Conference championships	2	2	2	2	2
3. Postseason appearances	2	2	2	2	2
B. Tier II sports (NCAA sports)					
1. Winning percentage	50	50	50	50	50
2. Conference championships	4	4	4	4	4
V. Media Relations					
A. Media coverage					
1. National spots	1	2	3	3	3
2. Regional spots	2	3	4	4	4
3. State	2	3	4	4	4
4. Local	2	3	4	4	4
B. Awards for Tier I media guides					
1. National (COSIDA) (Top 25)	1	1	1	1	1
2. Regional (Top 25%)	2	2	2	2	2
3. Conference (Top 3)	3	3	3	3	3
C. Staffing					
1. Internet/computer employee	1	1	1	1	1
VI. Business Administration					
A. Reduction in equipment costs (of Year 0 costs)	20%	25%	30%	30%	30%
B. Increase staff					
1. Volleyball assistant	0	1	1	2	2
2. Senior women's administrator	0	0	0	0	1
3. Women's basketball paid third assistant	0	1	1	1	1
4. Secretaries	0	1	1	2	2
5. Baseball paid second assistant	0	0	0	1	1

AREAS/OBJECTIVES	Year 1	Year 2	Year 3	Year 4	Year 5
C. Additional funding					
1. Personnel					
2. Recruiting					
3. Equipment					
4. Travel					
5. Salaries					
6. Advertising					
D. Varsity Club	50	100	150	200	250

ACTION PLAN

AREA: I. Academics

OBJECTIVES:	Year 1	Year 2	Year 3	Year 4	Year 5
A. GPA	2.65	2.70	2.75	2.80	2.85

STRATEGIES:
1. Recruit strong academic student-athletes
2. Increase tutor bank for student-athletes
3. Improve advising for class scheduling
4. Increase in center for counseling

Action	Person Responsible	Resources Required	Date Started	Date Completed
1. Identify and pursue strong academic student-athletes	Coach and Admissions	No additional	Year 1	Ongoing
2. Hire tutors for general ed classes	Academic Coordinator, Tutor Support	$4,000	Year 2	Ongoing
3. Hire qualified advisors	Academic Coordinator	$2,000	Year 3	Ongoing
4. Educate staff in counseling	Academic Coordinator	$1,000	Year 2	Ongoing

ACTION PLAN

AREA: I. Academics

OBJECTIVES:	Year 1	Year 2	Year 3	Year 4	Year 5
B. Graduation rate (percent of those who declare majors)	35	38	41	44	50

STRATEGIES:
1. Develop career counseling and testing
2. Begin a job fair for student-athletes
3. Educate coaches on importance of graduation
4. Develop counseling and motivational meetings for student-athletes

Action	Person Responsible	Resources Required	Date Started	Date Completed
1. Create a career division in Counseling Center	Academic Coordinator	$10,000	Year 4	Ongoing
2. Organize area businesses to recruit student-athletes for careers and educate	Athletic Director, Academic Coordinator	$1,000	Year 3	Annually
3. Have periodic meetings with coaches	Academic Coordinator, Compliance Coordinator	$2000 None	Year 3 Year 2	Ongoing Ongoing
4. Organize meetings with student-athletes to encourage completion of degree: use extra resources as available	Academic Coordinator	$500	Year 2	Ongoing

ACTION PLAN

AREA: I. Academics

OBJECTIVES:	Year 1	Year 2	Year 3	Year 4	Year 5
C. Expansion of Academic Learning Center					
1. Full-time counselors	0	0	1	1	2
2. Additional computers	4	2	2	2	2
3. Increase funding for additional resources by 10 percent each year	0	1,000	1,500	2,000	2,500
4. Life skills/Community Service Program	1	2	3	3	3

STRATEGIES:

1. Turn graduate assistant positions into full-time appointments
2. Add two new desktop or laptop computers each year to the Counseling Center
3. Increase learning and research resources available for student-athletes

Action	Person Responsible	Resources Required	Date Started	Date Completed
1a. Begin institutional funding of athletics academic area	CEO/Academic Coordinator	$36,000	Year 3	Year 4
1b. Hire a qualified counselor	Compliance Coordinator	$18,000	Year 3	Ongoing
2. Identify specific needs and request bids	Academic Coordinator, Compliance Coordinator	$2,000 $4,000	Year 3 Year 3	Ongoing Ongoing
3a. Identify research needs of student-athletes	Academic Coordinator	$500	Year 3	Ongoing
3b. Purchase resource material for computers and resource library in Counseling Center	Academic Coordinator	$1,000	Year 2	Ongoing

ACTION PLAN

AREA: II. Compliance

OBJECTIVES:	Year 1	Year 2	Year 3	Year 4	Year 5
A. Increase percentage of minority student-athletes	30%	32%	34%	35%	35%

STRATEGIES:

    1. Identify more potential minority student-athletes and recruit them to attend university

Action	Person Responsible	Resources Required	Date Started	Date Completed
1a. Contact state high school coaches	Coaches	None	Year 1	Ongoing
1b. Contact minority students on campus and encourage them to participate in athletics	Coaches	None	Year 1	Ongoing
1c. Identify regional high schools with large minority populations and encourage all coaches to visit and evaluate all these schools	Coaches and Athletic Director	None	Year 1	Ongoing

ACTION PLAN

AREA: II. Compliance

OBJECTIVES:	Year 1	Year 2	Year 3	Year 4	Year 5
B. Increase number of female student-athletes	42%	45%	48%	51%	54%

STRATEGIES:
1. Increase recruiting expenditures for women's teams
2. Require coaches to use maximum scholarships available
3. Increase number of coaches in women's athletics

Action	Person Responsible	Resources Required	Date Started	Date Completed
1. Provide additional resources for each women's sport	CEO and Athletic Director	$29,000	Year 2	Ongoing
2. Monitor recruitment and walk-on process to ensure maximum utilization of resources	Athletic Director	NONE	Year 1	Ongoing
3. Provide salaries to women's athletics to hire maximum number of coaches allowed by NCAA	CEO and Athletic Director	?	Year 2	Ongoing

ACTION PLAN

AREA: II. Compliance

OBJECTIVES:	Year 1	Year 2	Year 3	Year 4	Year 5
C. Increase funding for women's athletics	$44,000	$88,000	$132,000	$176,000	$220,000

STRATEGIES:
1. Increase salaries of current coaches to equal men's sports
2. Add coaches to maximum number allowed by the NCAA
3. Increase operating expenses

Action	Person Responsible	Resources Required	Date Started	Date Completed
1. Increase coaches' salaries of women's sports	CEO and Athletic Director	$45,000	Year 2	Ongoing
2. Increase number of coaches in women's basketball, volleyball, and golf	CEO and Athletic Director	$75,000	Year 2	Ongoing
3. Increase revenue for recruiting, equipment, and travel	CEO and Athletic Director	$100,000	Year 2	Ongoing

ACTION PLAN

AREA: II. Compliance

OBJECTIVES:	Year 1	Year 2	Year 3	Year 4	Year 5
D. Increase number of minority and female staff members	0	1	2	3	3

STRATEGIES:

1. Hire staff to assist with compliance and NCAA sport responsibilities

Action	Person Responsible	Resources Required	Date Started	Date Completed
1a. Commit to the strategy and provide funding for position	CEO and Athletic Director	$20,000	Year 2	Year 2
1b. Initiate a national search for qualified female candidates to serve this role	Compliance Coordinator	$2,500	Year 2	Year 2

ACTION PLAN

AREA: III. Marketing

OBJECTIVES:	Year 1	Year 2	Year 3	Year 4	Year 5
A. Season ticket sales					
1. Basketball	1,300	1,400	1,500	1,600	1,700

STRATEGIES:

1. Package men's and women's basketball together
2. Create a menu of affordable ticket options
3. Produce quality brochures to market the product
4. Renew existing customers
5. Identify primary and secondary target markets to cultivate new customers
6. Advertise the product

Action	Person Responsible	Resources Required	Date Started	Date Completed
1. Make a decision and commitment to combine the season tickets for men's and women's basketball	CEO, Athletic Director, Assistant Athletic Director	None	Immediately	N/A
2a. Study what the competition is doing, then develop and price our menu of options accordingly	Marketing Staff	Time	Nov. 1	Ongoing
2b. Make recommendations to Athletic Director, check with head basketball coaches, present to University President's office for final approval	Assistant Athletic Director	None	May 15	N/A
3. Graphics co. and the University Print Shop will produce the brochure under the direction of the Athletic Marketing Office	Marketing	Budget $	when schedules are set	Sept. 15
4a. Establish deadlines for renewal orders (Aug. 15 with Sept. 1 as final cutoff)	Marketing	Budget $	June 1	June 15
4b. Design and print a renewal card (by June 15)	Marketing	Budget $	June 1	June 15

Action	Person Responsible	Resources Required	Date Started	Date Completed
4c. Draft and print letter from head basketball coach(es) (by June 15)	Marketing and Coach	Letterhead	June 1	June 15
4d. Mail renewal card and letter to current customers (by July 1)	Marketing	$ for postage and time	July 1	July 1
4e. Follow up (phone and reminder letter) with all customers not yet renewed by August 15	Marketing	$ for postage and time	August 15	Sept. 1
4f. Cut off renewal process on 9/1	Marketing	N/A	N/A	Sept. 1
5a. Brainstorming session to identify both primary and secondary target markets	Marketing	Time	Continuous	
5b. Primary markets would include local area alumni, sports (basketball) fans, families of kids attending our summer basketball camps, business and/or professionals looking for opportunities to treat employees or entertain customers				
6a. Establish trade agreements when possible with both electronic (TV and radio) and print (newspapers and magazines) media outlets	Marketing	Time	Continuous	
6b. Create a line item in the university budget for advertising	Athletics Marketing	$	ASAP	N/A

ACTION PLAN

AREA: III. Marketing

OBJECTIVES:	Year 1	Year 2	Year 3	Year 4	Year 5
A. Season ticket sales					
2. Baseball	200	225	250	275	300

STRATEGIES:
1. Create a full menu of affordable ticket options
2. Produce quality brochures to market the product
3. Renew existing customers
4. Identify primary and secondary target markets to cultivate new customers
5. Advertise the product

Action	Person Responsible	Resources Required	Date Started	Date Completed
1a. Study what the competition is doing, then develop and price our menu of options accordingly	Marketing Staff	Time	Nov.	Ongoing
1b. Make recommendations to Athletic Director, check with head baseball coach, present to University President office for final approval	Marketing Director	None	May 15	N/A
2. Graphics co. and the University Print Shop will produce the brochure under the direction of the Athletic Marketing Office	Marketing	Budget $	When schedules are set	Nov. 15
3a. Establish deadlines for renewal orders (Jan. 1 with Jan. 15 as final cut-off)	Marketing	Budget $	June 1	June 15
3b. Design and print a renewal card (by Nov. 15)	Marketing	Budget $	June 1	Nov. 15
3c. Draft and print letter from head baseball coach (by Nov. 15)	Marketing and Coach	Letterhead	June 1	Nov. 15
3d. Mail renewal card and letter to current customers (by Dec. 1)	Marketing	$ for postage and time	Nov. 15	Dec. 1

Action	Person Responsible	Resources Required	Date Started	Date Completed
3e. Follow-up (phone and reminder letter) with all customers not yet re-newed by Jan. 1	Marketing	$ for post-age and time	Jan. 1	Jan. 15
3f. Cut off renewal process on Jan. 15	Marketing	N/A	N/A	Jan. 15
4. Brainstorming session to identify both primary and secondary target markets. Primary mar-kets would include local area alumni, sports (baseball) fans, families of kids attending our summer basketball camps, businesses, and/or professionals looking for opportunities to treat employees or entertain customers	Marketing	Time	Continuous	
5a. Establish trade agree-ments when possible with both electronic (TV and radio) and print (newspapers and maga-zines) media outlets	Marketing	Time	Continuous	
5b. Create a line item in the athletic marketing bud-get for advertising	University	$	ASAP	N/A

ACTION PLAN

AREA: III. Marketing

OBJECTIVES:	Year 1	Year 2	Year 3	Year 4	Year 5
A. Season ticket sales					
3. Volleyball	50	75	100	125	150

STRATEGIES:
1. Create a full menu of affordable ticket options
2. Produce quality brochures to market the product
3. Renew existing customers
4. Identify primary and secondary target markets to cultivate new customers
5. Advertise the product

Action	Person Responsible	Resources Required	Date Started	Date Completed
1a. Study what the competition is doing, then develop and price our own accordingly	Marketing Staff	Time	Nov.	Ongoing
1b. Make recommendations to Athletic Director, check with head volleyball coach, present to University President office for final approval	Assistant Athletic Director	None	May 15	N/A
2. Graphics co. and the University Print Shop will produce the brochure under the direction of the Athletic Marketing Office	Marketing	Budget $	When schedules are set	Aug. 1
3a. Establish deadlines for renewal orders (Aug. 1 with Aug. 15 as final cut-off)	Marketing	Budget $	June 1	June 15
3b. Design and print a renewal card (by May 15)	Marketing	Budget $	March 1	May 15
3c. Draft and print letter from head volleyball coach (by May 15)	Marketing and Coach	head	March 1	May 15
3d. Mail renewal card and letter to current customers (by June 1)	Marketing	$ for postage and time	May 15	June 1

Action	Person Responsible	Resources Required	Date Started	Date Completed
3e. Follow-up (phone and reminder letter) with all customers not yet renewed by Aug. 1	Marketing	$ for postage and time	July 15	August 1
3f. Cut off renewal process on Aug. 15	Marketing	N/A	N/A	August 15
4. Brainstorming session to identify both primary and secondary target markets. Primary markets would include local area alumni, sports (volleyball) fans, families of kids attending our summer basketball camps, Christian community, business and/or professionals looking for opportunities to treat employees or entertain customers	Marketing	Time	Continuous	
5a. Establish trade agreements when possible with both electronic (TV and radio) print (newspapers and magazines) media outlets	Marketing	Time	Continuous	
5b. Create a line item in the Athletic Marketing budget for advertising	University	$	ASAP	N/A

ACTION PLAN

AREA: III. Marketing

OBJECTIVES:	Year 1	Year 2	Year 3	Year 4	Year 5
A. Season ticket sales					
4. Soccer	100	125	150	200	250

STRATEGIES:

1. Create a full menu of affordable ticket options
2. Produce quality brochures to market the product
3. Renew existing customers
4. Identify primary and secondary target markets to cultivate new customers
5. Advertise the product

Action	Person Responsible	Resources Required	Date Started	Date Completed
1a. Study what the competition is doing, then develop and price our menu of options accordingly	Marketing Staff	Time	Nov.	Ongoing
1b. Make recommendations to Athletic Director, check with head Soccer coaches, present to University President office for final approval	Assistant Athletic Director	None	May 15	N/A
2. Graphics co. and the University Print Shop will produce the brochure under the direction of the Athletic Marketing Office	Marketing	Budget $	when schedules are set	Aug. 1
3a. Establish deadlines for renewal orders (Aug. 1 with Aug. 15 as final cut-off	Marketing	Budget $	June 1	June 15
3b. Design and print a renewal card (by May 15)	Marketing	Budget $	May 1	May 15
3c. Draft and print letter from head soccer coach (by May 15)	Marketing and Coach	Letterhead	May 1	June 1
3d. Mail renewal card and letter to current customers (by June 1)	Marketing	$ for postage and time	May 15	June 1

Action	Person Responsible	Resources Required	Date Started	Date Completed
3e. Follow-up (phone and reminder letter) with all customers not yet renewed by Aug. 1	Marketing	$ for postage and time	June 15	Aug. 1
3f. Cut off renewal process on Aug. 15	Marketing	N/A	N/A	Aug. 15
4. Brainstorming session to identify both primary and secondary target markets. Primary markets would include local area alumni, sports (soccer) fans, families of kids attending our summer basketball camps, Christian community, businesses, and/or professionals looking for opportunities to treat employees or entertain customers	Marketing	Time	Continuous	
5a. Establish trade agreements when possible with both electronic (TV and radio) and print (newspapers and magazines) media outlets	Marketing	Time	Continuous	
5b. Create a line item in the Athletics Marketing budget for advertising	University	$	ASAP	N/A

ACTION PLAN

AREA: III. Marketing

OBJECTIVES:	Year 1	Year 2	Year 3	Year 4	Year 5
B. Group sales					
1. Basketball	5,000	5,500	6,000	6,500	7,000
2. Baseball	200	250	300	350	400
3. Volleyball	50	100	150	200	250
4. Soccer	200	250	300	350	400

STRATEGIES:
1. Identify target markets for group sales
2. Hire additional personnel to handle
3. Create flyers/publications (brochures) to market group events

Action	Person Responsible	Resources Required	Date Started	Date Completed
1a. Churches	Marketing	Time and $ for addition- al things	Continuous	
1b. Civic	Marketing	Time and $ for addition- al things	Continuous	
1c. Corporations	Marketing	Time and $ for addition- al things	Continuous	
2. Make commitment that this is priority enough to hire staff person(s) to handle	University	$20,000	ASAP	N/A
3. Work with graphics co. and University Print Shop to design and print group event brochures	Marketing	Time and $ for printing	ASAP	N/A

ACTION PLAN

AREA: III. Marketing

OBJECTIVES:	Year 1	Year 2	Year 3	Year 4	Year 5
D. Attendance (per game)					
1. Basketball					
a. Overall	5,000	5,250	5,500	5,750	6,000
b. University students, faculty, and staff	1,500	1,600	1,700	1,800	1,900
2. Baseball					
a. Overall	350	400	450	500	550
b. University students, faculty, and staff	50	75	100	125	150
3. Volleyball					
a. Overall	250	300	350	375	450
b. University students, faculty, and staff	200	225	250	275	300
4. Soccer					
a. Overall	300	350	400	450	500
b. University students, faculty, and staff	150	175	200	225	250
5. Ticket revenue overall					
a. New season tickets	$17,250	$15,550	$17,050	$18,600	$20,300
b. Group sales	$12,950	$14,350	$15,750	$17,150	$18,550
c. Game day sales	$18,000	$19,000	$20,000	$21,000	$22,000
d. Total	$48,200	$48,900	$52,800	$56,750	$60,850

STRATEGIES:
1. Renew current season ticket customers
2. Cultivate new season ticket customers
3. Develop group sales program
4. Develop corporate "Promotional Nights" program
5. Bring in special guest entertainment (the mascot, etc.)
6. Win! Win! Win!
7. Hire additional staff

Action	Person Responsible	Resources Required	Date Started	Date Completed
1. Explained in season ticket sales Objective A	Marketing	Time and $ for additional staff, postage, printing, advertising	Continuous	
2. "	"	"		"

3. Objective B	"	"	"
4a. Sell balcony tickets for basketball to a company for a set price, then distribute vouchers for the event at sponsor locations	"	"	"
4b. Promotional item (provided by sponsor) given away to fans attending game	"	"	"
5. Select dates and celebrity entertainers desired and book them. Advertise!	"	$ to hire entertainer (celebrity)	"
6. Local will follow winning programs . . . we have to win!	Coaches and Student Athletes	$ to recruit better athletes and keep coaches	
7. If we want to improve the quality of something, it is going to cost us something. This is an investment!	Management	$	

ACTION PLAN

AREA: III. Marketing

OBJECTIVES:	Year 1	Year 2	Year 3	Year 4	Year 5

E. Sponsorship sales
   (cash and trade)

1. Basketball	200,000				
2. Baseball	60,000				
3. Volleyball					
4. Soccer					

STRATEGIES:
1. Maintain (renew) all current corporate partnerships
2. Identify targets for developing new corporate partner relationships
3. Purchase/create new signage and sponsorship opportunities

Action	Person Responsible	Resources Required	Date Started	Date Completed
1a. Maintain competitive menu of sponsor opportunities	Athletic Director	Time		Continuous
1b. Keep our sponsors informed through newsletters. Make them feel included.	Marketing	Time and $ for postage and printing		Continuous
2a. Review who is sponsoring the competition	Marketing	Time		Continuous
2b. Set up appointments to introduce new programs to these potential sponsors	Athletic Director	Time		Continuous
3a. Purchase additional signage tables, scoreboard, marque	University/ Marketing	$		Continuous
3b. Create new sponsorship ideas like the CITGO starting line-ups, halftime reports, etc.	Marketing	Time and creative thought		Continuous

ACTION PLAN

AREA: III. Marketing

OBJECTIVES:	Year 1	Year 2	Year 3	Year 4	Year 5
F. Merchandising	10,000	20,000	30,000	40,000	50,000

STRATEGIES:
1. Gain "on campus" sales rights for university apparel
2. Purchase beginning inventory of merchandise
3. Sell at volleyball, basketball, baseball games (maybe even soccer)
4. Catalog sales
5. Internet sales

Action	Person Responsible	Resources Required	Date Started	Date Completed
1. Renegotiate existing contract with Follett Bookstores	Athletic Director		ASAP	ASAP
2a. Select and purchase inventory	Marketing	$5,000	By Sept. 1	N/A
2b. Reorder when sold out	Marketing	$?	as needed	N/A
2c. Hire personnel to Management	Marketing	$?	By Sept. 1	N/A
3. See 2c action	Marketing	"	"	"
4a. Develop an inventory to manage catalog sales	Marketing	$	"	"
4b. Toll-free number needs to be established				
4c. Design and print catalog				
5a. Develop new athletics homepage	Marketing/ Media Relations	Time and $ to hire personnel	"	"
5b. See actions 4a and 4b	"			

ACTION PLAN

AREA: III. Marketing

OBJECTIVES:	Year 1	Year 2	Year 3	Year 4	Year 5
G. Golden Badge Club development	75,000	100,000	125,000	150,000	175,000

STRATEGIES:

1. Maintain current donors
2. Develop new memberships from identified target markets
3. Establish new innovative fund-raising events
4. Create an incentive plan to increase giving levels

Action	Person Responsible	Resources Required	Date Started	Date Completed
1. Say thank you, make them feel appreciated and part of the team; keep them informed through consistent, quality communication	Marketing	Time and $	NOW!	NEVER!
2a. Identify primary targets	"	Time		
2b. Create informative brochure promoting the organization and benefits of becoming a member: mail to targets!	"	Time and $	By Aug. 1	N/A
2c. See 2b action				
2d. Form committee to assist in membership drive	"	Time	NOW!	NEVER!
3a. Golf tour(s) in local and around USA in key alumni cities	"	Time and $	Future	?
3b. Auctions	"	Time	"	?
4a. Form committee to brainstorm	"	"	"	?
4b. Review what the competition is doing	"	"	"	?
4c. Like our idea to package season tickets into membership . . . parking, priority seating, etc.	"	"	Continuous	

ACTION PLAN

AREA: III. Marketing

OBJECTIVES:	Year 1	Year 2	Year 3	Year 4	Year 5
H. Capital campaign	200,000	210,000	215,000	N/A	N/A

STRATEGIES:
1. Seek donations from community sponsors in the business sector, foundations, and individual donors.
2. Upgrade facilities to be competitive with similar institutions

Action	Person Responsible	Resources Required	Date Started	Date Completed
1. Identify potential sponsors and seek major contributions	Athletic Director	Minimal	Under-way	Ongoing
2a. Review facilities/determine needs	Athletic Director	See plan IV	Under-way	Ongoing
2b. Raise needed funds	Assistant Athletic Director Marketing, University Development GEC			

ACTION PLAN

AREA: III. Marketing

OBJECTIVES:	Year 1	Year 2	Year 3	Year 4	Year 5
I. Additional Staff	1	2	1	0	1

STRATEGIES:

   1. Hire additional staff to assist in ticket sales (season and group), merchandise sales, and sponsorship sales

Action	Person Responsible	Resources Required	Date Started	Date Completed
1a. Identify qualified candidates	Athletic Director Assistant Athletic Director	Minimal $ (pay base salary and commission)	ASAP	Ongoing
1b. Interview candidates	Athletic Director Assistant Athletic Director			
1c. Delegate tasks				
1d. Oversee operations				

ACTION PLAN

AREA: III. Marketing

OBJECTIVES:	Year 1	Year 2	Year 3	Year 4	Year 5
J. Broadcast Affiliates					
1. Men's basketball	100%	100%	100%	100%	100%
2. Women's basket-ball	25%	50%	75%	100%	100%
3. Baseball	50%	50%	75%	75%	100%

STRATEGIES:

1. Broadcast men's basketball, women's basketball, and baseball games on radio affiliate(s) in local market
2. Broadcast a selected number of men's basketball, women's basketball, and baseball games on local TV, some broadcasts will be live and some tape-delayed
3. Develop a network of radio affiliates in markets around the state

Action	Person Responsible	Resources Required	Date Started	Date Completed
1a. Negotiate radio contracts for marketing women's basketball and baseball with local area broadcast affiliate(s)	Athletic Director, Assistant Athletic Director, Head Coach	$ to purchase air time and pay talent fee	Under-way	Ongoing
1b. Select broadcast team for each sport				
1c. Select specific games to be broadcast for women's basketball and baseball				
2a. Select broadcast team for each sport				
2b. Select specific games to be broadcast for each sport				
3a. Identify potential markets for expanded radio network				
3b. Explore interest with affiliates in those markets				

ACTION PLAN

AREA: III. Marketing

OBJECTIVES:	Year 1	Year 2	Year 3	Year 4	Year 5
K. Community relations (Speaker's Bureau)			See next page		

STRATEGIES:

1. Our coaches, athletes, mascot, and administrators should do at least one community event each month for a school or charity organization. Our coaches and administrators should be booked for speaking engagements at civic groups, schools, churches, charity events, and other community relations activities as often as possible. Certain months will be busier than others (two or three engagements per week), while other times will be very light such as one per month.

Action	Person Responsible	Resources Required	Date Started	Date Completed
1a. Contact all area civic groups, schools, churches, and charity organizations to inform them of our interest in scheduling our coaches, student-athletes, mascot, etc. to speak at and/or assist with their upcoming functions	Athletic Director, Assistant Athletic Director, Marketing Assistant, Coaches	Time to call	In process	Ongoing
1b. Follow up and market ourselves				

ACTION PLAN

AREA: IV. Competition

OBJECTIVES:	Year 1	Year 2	Year 3	Year 4	Year 5
A. Tier I Sports (men's basketball, women's basketball, volleyball, baseball)					
1. Winning percentage	60	62.5	65	67.5	67.5
2. Conference championships	2	2	2	2	2
3. Postseason appearances	2	2	2	2	2
B. Tier II Sports (NCAA sports)					
1. Winning percentage	50	50	50	50	50
2. Conference championships	4	4	4	4	4

STRATEGIES:
1. Maintain quality coaches
2. Upgrade recruiting
3. Keep players eligible
4. Improve facilities
5. Play appropriate schedules
6. Maintain proper budget

Action	Person Responsible	Resources Required	Date Started	Date Completed
1. Hire, motivate, and properly compensate coaches	Athletic Director	Variable depending on market		Ongoing
2. Find and sign better student athletes	Coaches	Some additional (see Plan VI C)		Ongoing
3. Provide academic support and counseling monitor progress of student athletes	Academic	Some additional (see Plan I D)	Underway	Ongoing
4. Raise $1.2 million to be paid over five-year period for new facilities and renovations	Athletic Director	$1.2 million	Year 1	Year 2

Action	Person Responsible	Resources Required	Date Started	Date Completed
5. Schedule opponents to achieve desired winning percentage, to promote ticket sales, to maintain high RPI and to prepare for Conference Championships	Coaches and Athletic Director	Some additional (see Plan VI C)	Underway	Ongoing
6. Increase funding to support actions 1 through 5	University Development, Athletic Director, Assistant Athletic Director, Marketing, Ticket Office, GEC	Some additional (see Plans I D, III H, VI C)		Ongoing

ACTION PLAN

AREA: V. Media Relations

OBJECTIVES:	Year 1	Year 2	Year 3	Year 4	Year 5
A. Media coverage					
1. National spots	1	2	3	3	3
2. Regional spots	2	3	4	4	4
3. State	2	3	4	4	4
4. Local	2	3	4	4	4

STRATEGIES:

1. Inform national media of key athletic events, competitive teams, and impressive athletes
2. Promote university athletics in surrounding states
3. Keep in close contact with all state outlets
4. Let local media know about upcoming events, results of completed events, conference standing, ideas for features

Action	Person Responsible	Resources Required	Date Started	Date Completed
1. Send media guides, releases, and fax scores to national media	Sports Information Director/ Assistant	Existing	Year 1	Ongoing
2. Make sure AP puts releases on regional wire	Sports Information Director/ Assistant	Existing	Year 1	Ongoing
3. Send releases, visit with state outlets	Sports Information Director/ Assistant	Existing	Year 1	Ongoing
1,2,3. Send hometown releases (features or feature ideas) to athletes' hometowns	Sports Information Director/ Assistant	Existing	Year 1	Ongoing
4. Media guides, releases, enthusiastic dialogue with local media outlets	Sports Information Director/ Assistant	Existing	Year 1	Ongoing

ACTION PLAN

AREA: V. Media Relations

OBJECTIVES:	Year 1	Year 2	Year 3	Year 4	Year 5
B. Awards for Tier I media guides					
1. National (COSIDA)	1 guide in top 25	same	same	same	same
	2 guides in top 25	same	same	same	same
2. Regional COSIDA)	3 guides in top 3	same	same	same	same
3. Conference					

STRATEGIES:
1. Fulfill COSIDA contest guidelines to the best of budget
2. Fulfill COSIDA contest guidelines to the best of budget
3. Fulfill conference guidelines for media guides

Action	Person Responsible	Resources Required	Date Started	Date Completed
1. Identify areas in media guides that need to be improved upon and make needed changes, Additions	Sports Information Director/ Assistant	Computers	Year 1	Ongoing
2. Same as #1				
3. Know conference guidelines . . . improve every year on existing guides	Sports Information Director/ Assistant	Computers, printing budget	Year 1	Ongoing

ACTION PLAN

AREA: V. Media Relations

OBJECTIVES:	Year 1	Year 2	Year 3	Year 4	Year 5
C. Staffing					
1. Internet/computer employee	1	1	1	1	1

STRATEGIES:
  1. Create athletics department home page for Internet
  2. Maintain athletics department computers—troubleshoot, install programs, upgrade, perform regular maintenance

Action	Person Responsible	Resources Required	Date Started	Date Completed
1. Hire Information Systems person to create Internet page	Athletic Director/ Sports Information Director	At least $30,000	Year 1	Ongoing
2. Be available to Athletic department personnel to maintain computers	Information systems employee	$2,500	Year 1	Ongoing

ACTION PLAN

AREA: VI. Business Administration

OBJECTIVES:	Year 1	Year 2	Year 3	Year 4	Year 5
A. Reduction in equipment costs	20%	25%	30%	30%	30%

STRATEGIES:
  1. Increase amount of free products given by vendors
  2. Order equipment in large quantities for lower cost
  3. Educate coaches on which products are best value
  4. Have a rotating system on number of products purchased each year

Action	Person Responsible	Resources Required	Date Started	Date Completed
1. Help coaches get contracts with sporting good companies	Business Administration	None	Year 1	Ongoing
2. Have coaches buy same brands and purchase at one time	Business Administration	None	Year 1	Ongoing
3. Meet with coaches to compare brands and prices	Business Administration	None	Year 1	Ongoing
4. Alternate buying patterns	Business Administration and coaches	None	Year 1	Ongoing

ACTION PLAN

AREA: VI. Business Administration

OBJECTIVES:	Year 1	Year 2	Year 3	Year 4	Year 5
B. Increase staff					
1. Volleyball Assistant	0	1	1	2	2
2. Senior women's administration	0	0	0	0	1
3. Women's Basketball Paid Third Assistant	0	1	1	1	1
4. Secretaries	0	1	1	2	2
5. Baseball Paid Assistant	0	0	0	1	1

STRATEGIES:
1. Comply with Title IX and NCAA Gender Equity guidelines
2. Increase budget to to enhance athletic department effectiveness
3. Increase budget to improve overall quality of baseball program

Action	Person Responsible	Resources Required	Date Started	Date Completed
1. Review Title IX/gender equity objectives for compliance	Athletic Director/ Assistant Athletic Director		Year 2	Ongoing
2. Identify departments that need additional staffing	Compl. and Marketing		Year 2	Ongoing
3. Evaluate top twenty-five baseball programs	Athletic Director		Year 3	Ongoing

ACTION PLAN

AREA: VI. Business Administration

OBJECTIVES: Year 1   Year 2   Year 3   Year 4   Year 5

C. Additional Funding
   1. Personnel
   2. Recruiting
   3. Equipment
   4. Travel
   5. Salaries
   6. Advertising

ACTION PLAN

AREA: VI. Business Administration

OBJECTIVES:	Year 1	Year 2	Year 3	Year 4	Year 5
D. Varsity Club	50	100	150	200	250

STRATEGIES:
1. Build database of alumni
2. Begin hall of fame
3. Alumni golf tournament
4. Raise funds

Action	Person Responsible	Resources Required	Date Started	Date Completed
1. Call Alumni Association and former players for current addresses	Business Manager	None	Year 1	Ongoing
2. Select and induct members	Business Manager	$1,000	Year 1	Ongoing
3. Invite alumni to play in golf tournament during homecoming weekend	Business Manager	None	Year 1	Ongoing
4. Send quarterly news-letter with application to join varsity club	Business Manager	$500	Year 1	Ongoing

Appendix D

Employee Evaluation and Development Form

University of Maryland Athletics
PERFORMANCE REVIEW
AND DEVELOPMENT PROCESS
SETTING EXPECTATIONS AND FINAL APPRAISAL
EMPLOYEE FORM

Employee Name: Supervisor:
ED Number: Period Covering:
Job Title: Date of Review:
Division/Dept: Section/Unit:

Expectation Setting Meeting Held and Job Priorities Discussed:

_____   _____
Supervisor's Signature   Employee's Signature

Final Appraisal Meeting Held _____(Date)
Please check one: The employee and supervisor are [__ in agreement __ not in agreement] with the performance appraisal results. If not agreed, area(s) of disagreement are indicated below:

_____   _____
Supervisor's Signature   Employee's Signature

Reviewed by next higher level supervisor (or departmental designee):

_____   _____
Reviewer's Name (Please Print)   Reviewer's Signature

Note: The employee's signature does not necessarily indicate agreement with the performance appraisal result. The signature indicates only that the performance appraisal was held.

Outstanding   *Exemplary performance* in all areas of the job.

Exceeds   *Surpasses the standards* and established performance
Expectations   expectations in many important areas of the job.

Meets   Good performance. Consistently meets standards and
Expections   established performance expectations in important
                      areas of the job.

Below   Performance *does not meet expectations* in some im-
Expectations   portant areas of the job; below expected levels; im-
                      provement needed.

Unsatisfactory   Performance falls *below expectations in many areas* of
                      the job. Substantial improvement critical.

1. CUSTOMER SERVICE

Understanding the needs of internal and external customers; making special effort to be responsive in meeting their needs and in building customer satisfaction.

Definition of "Meets Expectations":

Outstanding	Exceeds Expectations	Meets Expectations	Below Expectations	Unsatisfactory
_____	_____	_____	_____	_____

Comments on Performance

2. COOPERATION AND TEAMWORK

Putting the group's success ahead of personal goals; sharing information and resources with others; giving timely response to requests made by others; promoting teamwork; exhibiting positive attitudes during times of change; taking on new tasks with enthusiasm and energy.

Definition of "Meets Expectations":

Outstanding	Exceeds Expectations	Meets Expectations	Below Expectations	Unsatisfactory
_____	_____	_____	_____	_____

Comments on Performance

3. COMMUNICATION SKILLS

Speaking clearly, concisely, and using words easily understood; exchanging ideas with others; listening to understand meaning; writing in a concise and appropriate manner.

Definition of "Meets Expectations":

Outstanding	Exceeds Expectations	Meets Expectations	Below Expectations	Unsatisfactory
_____	_____	_____	_____	_____

Comments on Performance

4. ATTENDANCE AND PUNCTUALITY

Coming to work regularly without excessive absences; maintaining assigned work schedules.

Definition of "Meets Expectations":

Outstanding	Exceeds Expectations	Meets Expectations	Below Expectations	Unsatisfactory
_____	_____	_____	_____	_____

Comments on Performance

5. QUALITY OF WORK

Completing work thoroughly, accurately, neatly, and according to specifications; producing output with minimal errors.

Definition of "Meets Expectations":

Outstanding	Exceeds Expectations	Meets Expectations	Below Expectations	Unsatisfactory
_____	_____	_____	_____	_____

Comments on Performance

6. QUANTITY OF WORK

Consistently producing a high volume of acceptable work; producing services or output quickly and efficiently.

Definition of "Meets Expectations":

Outstanding	Exceeds Expectations	Meets Expectations	Below Expectations	Unsatisfactory
_____	_____	_____	_____	_____

Comments on Performance

7. JOB KNOWLEDGE

Understanding job procedures, policies, and responsibilities; keeping up-to-date technically; acting as a resource person on whom others rely for assistance.

Definition of "Meets Expectations":

Outstanding	Exceeds Expectations	Meets Expectations	Below Expectations	Unsatisfactory
_____	_____	_____	_____	_____

Comments on Performance

8. SUPPLEMENTARY PERFORMANCE PROJECT/FACTOR

Definition:

Definition of "Meets Expectations":

Outstanding	Exceeds Expectations	Meets Expectations	Below Expectations	Unsatisfactory
_____	_____	_____	_____	_____

Comments on Performance

9. SUPPLEMENTARY PERFORMANCE PROJECT/FACTOR

Definition:

Definition of "Meets Expectations":

Outstanding	Exceeds Expectations	Meets Expectations	Below Expectations	Unsatisfactory
_____	_____	_____	_____	_____

Comments on Performance

10. SUPPLEMENTARY PERFORMANCE PROJECT/FACTOR

Definition:

Definition of "Meets Expectations":

Outstanding	Exceeds Expectations	Meets Expectations	Below Expectations	Unsatisfactory
_____	_____	_____	_____	_____

Comments on Performance

11. SUPPLEMENTARY PERFORMANCE PROJECT/FACTOR

Definition:

Definition of "Meets Expectations":

Outstanding	Exceeds Expectations	Meets Expectations	Below Expectations	Unsatisfactory
_____	_____	_____	_____	_____

Comments on Performance

DEVELOPMENT PLANS

To be completed by employee and supervisor together using information from previous sections

MAJOR STRENGTHS:
In which performance factors/ projects did the employee excel?

AREAS FOR IMPROVEMENT/ENHANCEMENT:

What performance factors/projects are in need of improvement or enhancement?

ACTION PLANS:

What actions should be taken by the employee and/or supervisor to improve the employee's performance and help achieve goal(s) during the next performance period?

	Action Plan	**Time Frame**
Employee:		
Supervisor:		

TRAINING PLANS

List the training actions that will be taken to improve performance weaknesses in the current job or to develop additional employee skills.

OVERALL RATING:

The supervisor must assign an overall rating to the employee's cumulative performance throughout the review cycle. The determination of the overall rating shall be consistent with the rating scale below.

Outstanding   *Exemplary performance* in all areas of the job.

Exceeds   *Surpasses the standards* and established performance
Expectations   expectations in many important areas of the job.

Meets   Good performance. Consistently meets standards and
Expections   established performance expectations in important
                 areas of the job.

Below   Performance *does not meet expectations* in some im-
Expectations   portant areas of the job; below expected levels; im-
                 provement needed.

Unsatisfactory   Performance falls *below expectations in many areas* of
                 the job. Substantial improvement critical.

Outstanding	Exceeds Expectations	Meets Expectations	Below Expectations	Unsatisfactory
_____	_____	_____	_____	_____

References

Bowden, William W., and Yow, Deborah A. 1996. "Survey of 260 Randomly Selected Adults Regarding Personal Goals and Enabling Objectives." Unpublished Research.

Bowden, William W., and Yow, Deborah A. 1998. "A Survey of NCAA Division I Athletic Programs in Regard to their Planning Procedures." Unpublished Research.

Bradford, David L., and Cohen, Allen R. 1984. *Managing for Excellence*. New York: John Wiley and Sons Press.

Bridges, Francis J., and Roquemore, Libby L. 1992. *Management for Athletic/Sport Administration*. Decatur, GA: ESM Books.

Dowling, William F., and Miller, Ernest C. (eds.). 1987. *Organization Dynamics*. New York: American Management Association.

Drucker, Peter. 1954. *The Practice of Management*. New York: Harper and Row.

Drucker, Peter. 1974. *Management: Tasks, Responsibilities and Practices*. New York: Harper and Row.

Migliore, R.H. 1983. *An MBO Approach to Long Range Planning*. Englewood Cliffs, NJ: Prentice-Hall.

Migliore, R.H., Yow, Deborah A., and Bowden, William W. 1998. "Planning Your Next (Management) Move: Winning Strategies." *Athletic Management* (February/March), pp. 19-22.

Oakley, Edward, and Krug, Douglas. 1991. *Enlightened Leadership*. New York: Simon and Schuster.

Thompson, Arthur A., Jr., and Strickland, A. J. 1986. *Strategy Formulation and Implementation*, Third edition. Plano, TX: Business Publications, Inc.

Yow, Deborah A. and Bowden, William W. 1998. "Planning Resources for Athletics Administration." College Park, MD: University of Maryland, Printed Lecture Notes.

Yow, Deborah A., Bowden, William W., and Humphrey, James H. 1998. "College Athletes Under Stress: Causes, Consequences, Coping." *Athletics Administration* (December), pp. 10-12.

Index

Order Your Own Copy of
This Important Book for Your Personal Library!

STRATEGIC PLANNING FOR COLLEGIATE ATHLETICS

_____ in hardbound at $39.95 (ISBN: 0-7890-0889-0)

_____ in softbound at $24.95 (ISBN: 0-7890-1057-7)

COST OF BOOKS_____

OUTSIDE USA/CANADA/
MEXICO: ADD 20%_____

POSTAGE & HANDLING_____
*(US: $3.00 for first book & $1.25
for each additional book)
Outside US: $4.75 for first book
& $1.75 for each additional book)*

SUBTOTAL_____

IN CANADA: ADD 7% GST_____

STATE TAX_____
*(NY, OH & MN residents, please
add appropriate local sales tax)*

FINAL TOTAL_____
*(If paying in Canadian funds,
convert using the current
exchange rate. UNESCO
coupons welcome.)*

☐ **BILL ME LATER:** ($5 service charge will be added)
(Bill-me option is good on US/Canada/Mexico orders only;
not good to jobbers, wholesalers, or subscription agencies.)

☐ Check here if billing address is different from
shipping address and attach purchase order and
billing address information.

Signature_____

☐ **PAYMENT ENCLOSED: $**_____

☐ **PLEASE CHARGE TO MY CREDIT CARD.**

☐ Visa   ☐ MasterCard   ☐ AmEx   ☐ Discover
☐ Diner's Club

Account #_____

Exp Date_____

Signature_____

Prices in US dollars and subject to change without notice.

NAME _____

INSTITUTION _____

ADDRESS _____

CITY _____

STATE/ZIP _____

COUNTRY _____ COUNTY (NY residents only) _____

TEL _____ FAX _____

E-MAIL_____
May we use your e-mail address for confirmations and other types of information? ☐ Yes   ☐ No

Order From Your Local Bookstore or Directly From
The Haworth Press, Inc.
10 Alice Street, Binghamton, New York 13904-1580 • USA
TELEPHONE: 1-800-HAWORTH (1-800-429-6784) / Outside US/Canada: (607) 722-5857
FAX: 1-800-895-0582 / Outside US/Canada: (607) 772-6362
E-mail: getinfo@haworthpressinc.com
PLEASE PHOTOCOPY THIS FORM FOR YOUR PERSONAL USE.

BOF96